Contents

Making birth easier

ANDREA ROBERTSON

ALLEN & UNWIN

First published 1990
Allen & Unwin Australia Pty Ltd
8 Napier Street, North Sydney NSW 2059 Australia

National Library of Australia
Cataloguing-in-Publication entry:

Robertson, Andrea.
Making birth easier.

Bibliography.
ISBN 0 04 44 2272 5.

1. Prenatal care. 2. Pregnancy. 3. Childbirth.
4. Natural Childbirth. I. Title

618.24

Set in 10/11.5 Garamond Book by Excel Imaging Pty Ltd
Printed by Australian Print Group, Maryborough, Vic.

Introduction

When I was having my children, 18 and 16 years ago, birth was an event that took place only in the hospital, with a doctor in attendance in a regimented, authoritarian labour ward. Even though I had worked in the health care system myself and had some idea of the way it functioned in other areas, I willingly gave myself over to it totally, became a regular patient, and lay down to take my 'medicine'. The notions of alternatives, choices and informed consent were unheard of at that time, and it was only after the second birth when I voiced some questions to my doctor, that I began to realise that consumers had little say in what happened to them at this most critical time in their lives.

I also realised that when a woman is pregnant, not only is she the consumer, so is the baby. I had to accept that the best spokesperson for my baby was me! My children's future health and well-being depended on my seeking and demanding the best possible care for myself during pregnancy, birth and in the early months of breastfeeding. I would have done this willingly had I known how, and it is only now, after years of involvement in the consumer movement that I have gained the insights I needed then. I believe that most mothers would willingly take more responsibility too if they knew how to go about it.

Childbirth education may have improved, midwives may be gaining a more visible profile in our hospitals and there are now numerous books, videos and magazines catering for the need of pregnant women for information. However, it continually surprises me that many women I see in pre-natal classes are still unaware of their legal rights, have little understanding of informed consent, and lack confidence in seeking second opinions or changing doctors. Some of this is due to the pregnant woman's need to be nurtured, and not to be fiercely assertive at this time. However, since women are notoriously protective of their babies then it should be natural for them to seek responsiblity for their babies right from the start.

It is difficult to take responsibility however, when you don't understand the system, are unfamiliar with the protocols and expectations of those caring for you, and are blissfully unaware of what questions to ask to obtain the information you need. This is the way many health care professionals would like it to stay. There is much talk of the importance of taking a consumer approach to health care, but how does one do this, given the climate favouring the status quo and the complexity and mystery of the health care system?

The first part of this book aims to give you the ground rules and options available to you as a pregnant parent. Spending time and energy on choosing a birth place, caregiver, support person, and labour management plan is worthwhile as it reduces anxieties during labour and this will lead to a quicker, safer and less painful birth. This section is directed to the mother and her partner, as you will both be involved in making these decisions together.

The second part of the book has been written primarily for the partner and support people of the mother during labour. Being in labour gives the mother permission to divorce herself totally from any need to be assertive, make decisions, interact with others or do anything other than work with her body to find the best way to give birth for her and the baby. This means that the support people must take over some of the responsibility, not by directing the labour, issuing instructions or dictating her actions, but by ensuring that she is protected from distraction, disturbance and anything that might interfere with the normal flow of hormones and behaviour that will characterise her labour.

The old image of the father 'coaching' his wife through labour contractions, urging her to breathe in structured ways, instructing her to 'sound out' the painful contractions is outdated. We now know that women need to be allowed to labour in their own way, with complete freedom to do whatever they feel is right at the time. This reassessment of the support person's role, however, has left many people, fathers included, bewildered about what they can do to make her labour more comfortable. The suggestions I have outlined are based on the idea that a labouring woman cannot be 'helped' to labour well, only provided with the right kind of support and environment that will allow her to use her instincts and hormones freely. Giving birth is up to her, we can only stand by and make sure she has our confidence and protection.

We have, as a community, largely forgotten what normal, unmedicated birth looks like. We have become so used to relying on machines, drips, injections and surgery that we have lost sight of the kind of birthing behaviour that women use to give birth easily and quickly. Today, having a natural physiologic birth (a birth as nature intends) means going against this tide of intervention. The sights and sounds of normal birth are unfamiliar to hospital midwives and doctors and will come as a surprise to them as well as to yourselves as support people. Keeping a level head in the face of an apparently overwhelming labour will take confidence and under-standing of the natural processes involved. I hope that after reading the section on 'What you will see' you will have the strength and conviction to trust the mother to know her own needs during labour, and feel comfortable in giving her permission to behave naturally.

I would suggest that you read this book alongside my other hand-book *Preparing for Birth*. It contains specific detail on the preg-nancy, labour, birth and post-partum period that you will need as a reference when asking questions, deciding on your options and making decisions. *Making Birth Easier* is intended as a companion volume and should be read alongside other sources of birth infor-mation. A suggested list of other titles to consult is at the end of this book.

Much of what is contained here is based on personal experiences of birth: my own, attending others', observations in hospital set-tings, and feedback from couples who have been through my pre-natal preparation programme. All of these have given me insights and invaluable experience, which I hope will inspire you to stick to your guns to make this coming birth whatever you want for yourselves.

Andrea Robertson
16 February 1990

PART 1

1

Choosing a birthplace

The environment in which a mother labours can have a strong effect on how she gives birth. To labour easily and quickly a mother must feel safe and secure, so choosing a place in which to give birth takes care and consideration.

There are several possible birth places that you should consider and discuss with your partner. Not all of these options may be available near where you live, but it may be worthwhile to travel to another town or city if the facilities there are what you want. It is important to consider your place of birth as early as possible in your pregnancy so that you have time to explore alternatives and make bookings.

When considering where you want to give birth, you will also need to discuss your thoughts with your midwife or doctor. They may be unable or unwilling to be with you at the birth if you choose to have your baby away from their normal setting. In this case, shopping around in your area may locate someone who will be able to help you, or you may choose an alternative birth place so that you can have the caregiver of your choice.

The hospital labour ward

This is the place the majority of women choose for the birth of their baby. In many cases, women don't actively make this choice, they just assume that the hospital is the traditional place for babies to be born or go there because that is where the doctors delivers babies.

- You know that the hospital is always available, with a full staff of midwives and doctors at your service.
- Everyone is welcome: a public hospital cannot turn you away. Private hospitals must be booked in advance.
- All the emergency equipment, medical facilities, drugs and technology are readily available. This is especially helpful when a problem occurs, as can sometimes happen.

- You will not be able to choose the midwives who care for you in labour and you may not be able to meet them in advance. A private doctor will arrive for the birth, and hospital patients will usually have their baby delivered by the midwife on duty. In a teaching hospital, student midwives and doctors may also assist and deliver the baby as part of their training.
- Early discharge schemes are available in some hospitals. The mother can choose to stay in hospital after the birth or to go home after a few hours, with a midwife who will visit in the first week.

Many hospitals today have taken some steps towards humanising the environment, by providing wallpaper, soft furnishings and a more liberal attitude towards labouring women's needs. This helps to make the place less forbidding and more comfortable, which can make labour easier.

Birth centres

These have developed in response to consumer demand for a home-like birthing place within a hospital setting.

- A birth centre has a room or series of rooms set up like a normal bedroom, usually with bathroom and kitchen facilities and often a lounge area.
- It is staffed by a team of selected midwives who provide the pregnancy care (sometimes on a share basis with a private doctor) and help at the birth.
- A birth centre emphasises normal, physiologic management of the labour and birth without drugs or medical interventions. Should a complication arise, then transfer is made to the normal labour room facilities nearby.
- The centre allows complete freedom to choose birth companions, labour and delivery positions and sibling involvement if desired.
- It may offer early discharge with a midwife to visit you at home in the early days after the birth. This will avoid a stay in the hospital's post-natal section, which however is an attractive option for some mothers, especially if they have other children at home.

Most birth centres have a list of conditions under which a mother will be unable to use the facilities, and must use the labour room instead. Although these conditions are designed to make the birth safer in a birth centre, many of them are questionable, such as age limitations on the mother, previous obstetric complications and time limits on the pregnancy. When considering a birth centre, you should ask about these exclusion criteria and try to assess the staff's flexibility in applying them.

Birthing rooms

As a cheaper alternative to birth centres, with their special staff and facilities, many hospitals have set up birthing rooms within the normal labour ward complex.

- A birthing room is located within the normal labour ward area.
- It has soft furnishings, usually including a regular single or double bed rather than a labour room delivery bed. En-suite facilities may be available.
- The room has the normal labour room equipment but it is screened or concealed to give the room a less clinical atmosphere. This may mean the mother does not need to be transferred if a problem occurs.
- It is staffed by midwives who are not specially selected, but work in the whole labour room area. The doctor will usually deliver the baby rather than the midwife, unless the mother specifically requests midwifery care.
- A birthing room may be available for any mother having a baby, but some hospitals apply restrictions so that only known low-risk mothers may use the room. By doing this, the parents and staff are encouraged to regard the birthing room as an alternative to the regular labour room, with a special emphasis on normal, physiologic birth.
- It may offer early discharge with midwife home visits, otherwise the mother will stay in the regular post-natal area.

Homebirth

As the importance of the birth environment has become more widely recognised, an increasing number of women have decided that the hospital setting feels altogether too uncomfortable and potentially threatening for birth, and as a result they have chosen to stay at home.

- Homebirth offers complete freedom to 'do your own thing' in labour according to your needs and wishes. Privacy is easily obtained and respected.

- You have the freedom to choose birthing companions and caregivers, who can freely provide support and assistance as needed.
- There is no possibility of medical intervention or pain relieving drugs being available or used. Many women enjoy the peace of mind this allows.
- There are no disruptions after the birth as the parents and baby stay together constantly and will not be separated for any reason.
- Post-natal care is provided by the midwife who visits during the first few days at home to help the mother establish breastfeeding and check on progress.

The choice of home as the place for your baby's birth will depend on the availability of a midwife who will care for you and the back up of a doctor in case a problem develops that requires medical assistance.

Post-natal care

When you give birth away from your own home, you will also need to consider your options about your post-natal stay in hospital. You may have the following alternatives:

Private rooms

Some hospitals have a limited number of private rooms which can be used by mothers who are privately insured. However, some hospitals have a policy of reserving these rooms for those mothers who are sick or who need extra care after the birth, such as after a caesarian section. In private hospitals, most of the post-natal rooms are either private or twin share and are available to everyone.

Full rooming-in

Many mothers like to have their babies with them all the time so that they can be cared for and fed in a flexible way. Some hospitals allow this option only if the mother has a private room, others leave it to the women in the shared ward to decide on a policy themselves. You should not, however, be penalised for wanting to have your baby with you all the time, as this is what the baby would prefer, so if there are some limitations you may like to consider going home early, moving to a room with other mothers who have their babies at night or convincing the other mothers in your room of your rights.

Shared rooms

These rooms usually have from two to four beds in each, and some may have their own en-suite facilities. Rooming-in options may vary according to your room-mates' preferences.

Partial rooming-in

In this case, the babies generally go to a centralised nursery at night, but are usually with their mothers during the day. Even if the baby is in the nursery at night, you can visit and feed the baby there as often as you need or wish, or instructions can be left that the baby is to be brought to you in bed for feeds when necessary. Some hospitals prefer that the babies return to the nursery during visiting time.

Motel-like accommodation

Minimum care post-natal accommodation where the mother and baby can stay together in a private room with either its own en-suite or nearby bathroom facilities is available in a few hospitals. This kind of accommodation is very popular and approximates being at home, but with help nearby and no cooking!

Early discharge and post-natal home visits

This is becoming more widely used in an effort to reduce hospital stays and help mothers establish their relationship with the baby in the comfort and privacy of their own home. Use of this service usually depends on the mother and baby being well, and living within a set distance from the hospital. A midwife calls daily in the first few days and extends her care if needed. Mothers using this service need to have good support from family and friends at home so that adequate rest and time with the baby can be achieved.

Visiting

In most hospitals today visiting times are flexible for partners and siblings. Some have an open visiting policy without special times (this can be very tiring for the new mother) and other still have set times for visitors.

Making the choice

Before you decide where you will give birth, enquire what options are available in your area. Sometimes it is worth travelling some distance to get the kind of care you feel will help you give birth easily. Finding the right people to help you during labour is also important, and this may influence your choice of birth place. It makes little sense to choose a birthplace where your midwife or doctor feel uncomfortable or are unable to practise, and there are many ways you can make a less than perfect environment more comfortable if necessary.

Visit the hospital, birth centre or birthing room and find out what it is like. You may be able to make an individual visit with your partner, or you may be asked to participate in a regular tour conducted by the staff. More than one visit may be needed.

When assessing the hospital's facilities and approach to birth, there are many questions you can ask. If the person conducting the labour ward tour does not work in the labour room, seek out a member of staff who works there, and is familiar with current policy and practice. You should also take the opportunity to visit the post- natal areas and the nursery, including intensive care. You need to know all about the hospital if you are to feel comfortable and familiar with its facilities.

Questions to ask when choosing a birthplace

- Whom may I have with me in labour? Are there any restrictions on the number of support people I can choose? Do I have to make special arrangements so my support people can attend?
- Will I be allowed to choose my own labour and birth positions and do whatever I feel will help me to labour comfortably? Do you have hot packs, bean bags, floor mats, and food and drink available, or should I bring my own?
- What routine procedures operate in this hospital? How often will I be examined, and what is the hospital policy regarding drugs?
- Will support people be excluded if the baby is born by caesarian section?
- Can I breastfeed immediately after the birth of the baby?
- Where are the shower and toilet that I can use during labour?
- Where can my support people have a break and make themselves a cup of tea?
- What do I need to bring to hospital? When do you suggest we come in during labour?

You should also take the opportunity to visit the intensive care nursery and the post-natal wards while you are at the hospital.

Although it is unlikely that your baby will need special care after it is born, it is helpful to have seen these places and so be better prepared for the equipment and activity that are found in the nursery areas.

When you are checking the post-natal wards, you can ask questions about your post-natal stay.

- What are the hospital's policies on rooming-in with the baby? Can I have the baby with me for the full 24 hours should I wish?
- Is breastfeeding supported? Are complementary feeds (formulas, glucose water, boiled water) suggested? Are babies brought to their mothers for night feeds if full rooming-in is not available?
- Is there a lactation consultant at the hospital?
- What arrangements are made for visitors?
- Will I be shown basic baby care, including bathing during the post-natal stay?
- Is there an early discharge program available, should I wish to use it? How soon can a mother leave hospital after the birth? Can the hospital provide any post-natal back-up services (phone contact, midwife to visit) should I wish to go home early?

2

Choosing professional help

One of the most important decisions you will have to make concerns choosing the person who will provide your midwifery or medical care during your pregnancy and birth. You want a professional adviser who communicates well and accepts your needs and whose judgement you feel you can trust. Your caregiver should understand that this is a special experience for you and that your needs are the most important consideration. You need to accept that in the unlikely event of a complication developing, your caregiver may need to make some professional decisions to ensure that you and your baby are as safe as possible. Since most of the time pregnancy and labour are normal, uncomplicated events, you should be in charge unless it is clear that special help is needed.

The midwife

A midwife is fully trained to provide pregnancy care, assistance at the birth and post-natal follow up. She (there are a few male midwives) is best equipped to guide you through the normal events of pregnancy and birth, whilst watching for those rare occasions when special help is needed, when she will summon a doctor for further assistance. Midwives have been the traditional carers of childbearing women for thousands of years, and their experience with a wide range of normal births and the unique needs of women give them special insights into ways of making birth easier and more satisfying.

The midwife usually works in a hospital, in the ante-natal wards, labour room area and in the post-natal wards. It is not usually possible to choose a midwife at the hospital, as they are rostered as a team, and the mother is cared for by the midwife on duty at the time.

In some areas midwives work independently from the hospital. Many of these care for women having home births, but some have arranged for visiting rights at the hospital, and can look after you in the same way as a doctor. These midwives provide pregnancy care, stay with you at home in the early part of labour, take you to hospital where they will assist you with the birth and then provide follow up care and support in your own home again shortly after the birth.

A home birth midwife provides a full service of ante-natal visits, assistance during labour and birth in your home and visits afterwards to check the progress of you and the baby. Should you need to be transferred to the hospital at some time during the labour or birth, your midwife will accompany you to the hospital and may continue to look after you there.

Independent midwives sometimes work in a group practice with other midwives or with a doctor, who provides medical back-up should it become necessary. Many midwives recommend that you make contact with a doctor at least twice during the pregnancy in case medical assistance is needed at the birth. Should this happen you would be helped by the doctor you have already met and who knows your medical history. The doctor may arrange the various pregnancy tests that are needed, if the midwife has not already done so.

Midwives charge fees according to the service they provide. Those employed by the hospital provide their services free of charge as part of the hospital's service. Some independent midwives provide a package which includes all visits, attendance at the birth and post-natal follow up for a set fee. Others bill for actual visits made with a standard fee for attendance at the birth. It can be difficult to obtain rebates for midwifery services at this time, but some private health funds do offer some cover. Check your health insurance policy on this point.

The doctor: the general practitioner

General practitioners provide maternity care in some communities. Although they are not fully qualified as obstetricians, these doctors are trained to provide medical care for mothers with normal pregnancies and births. Should an emergency occur, the GP will call in an obstetrician to assist. One advantage of GP care is that you probably already know the doctor and have established a relationship with him/her, and s/he will also provide further care for you and your family after the baby is born. General practitioners usually prefer to deliver babies in hospital, although some are available to do home births, often in conjunction with a midwife.

Most general practitioners charge the set fee specified by Medicare for pregnancy care, attendance at the birth and post-natal visits, but ask about any additional fees that may apply.

The obstetrician

Obstetricians are doctors who have specialised in the treatment and care of mothers and women with special problems or complicated pregnancies or labours. Some women prefer to have an obstetrician for ante-natal care and to deliver the baby even when there are no special problems, and are willing to pay for these services. While the obstetrician will see you for your ante-natal visits, the midwife in the labour ward will care for you in labour and call the doctor so that they arrive in time to deliver the baby. The obstetrician will visit you in hospital after the birth and see you again six weeks later for a check-up. Obstetricians work in hospital settings and are not available to do home births.

Obstetricians usually set their own fee scale for providing ante-natal care, delivering the baby and post-natal follow up. The standard Medicare rebate will be available but there could be a considerable gap that you will have to fund yourself unless you have private health insurance. In choosing an obstetrician you will automatically be charged for your hospital stay at the private rate, which will be covered if you have private health insurance.

The hospital outpatients clinic

Another option for pregnancy care is to attend the outpatients clinic at your local hospital. Not all hospitals provide this service, and some provide different types of clinics. At the clinic you will be under the nominal care of an obstetrician, but at your visits you will be seen by the clinic doctor, usually a registrar (a doctor in the final stages of training as an obstetrician), and you may see a different doctor each time. During labour, you will be attended by the hospital midwives who will usually deliver the baby. Sometimes, if there are trainee doctors or midwives at the hospital, they will deliver the baby under the guidance of the midwife or obstetrician.

Attending the outpatients clinic is free. Some hospitals use an appointment system but others have a general time, which may involve you in long waits.

In addition to the clinics described above, some hospitals are now providing midwives' clinics, staffed by a small team of midwives who see mothers for all the ante-natal care, and sometimes also deliver the baby. The emphasis is on wellness and continuity of care by the team.

Mothers planning to use a birth centre are usually offered shared pregnancy care by the midwives at the birth centre and either their own private doctor or the doctor at the outpatients clinic. Alternate visits are made to the birth centre midwives and the doctor, with the doctor arranging for any tests to be done. The birth is usually supervised by the midwife if the mother has been attending the outpatients clinic. If the mother has been seeing a private obstetrician, the birth may be managed by either the doctor or the midwife, depending on the mother's wishes.

When deciding what help you would prefer for the birth of your baby, you will first need to find out what choices are available in your area. Your local hospital can give you a list of doctors who attend births at the hospital. To find a midwife who practises independently you could contact the Community Health Centre, a Women's Health Centre, or one of the organisations that provide support and information for childbearing families or home births (try your telephone directory for your local Childbirth Education group).

Some women choose the obstetrician recommended by their general practitioner and others ask their friends to suggest doctors in the area. Making a decision about the right doctor for you takes time and is worth considering carefully. Although it is always possible to change doctors at any time, this can be more difficult if you need to make the change late in your pregnancy, as some of the more open-minded and flexible doctors limit the number of pregnant women they see each month to allow more time per patient.

Sometimes it is worthwhile visiting several doctors before you make up your mind. Ask your friends about their experiences, and in particular how willing their doctor was to accommodate specific requests for management of the labour and birth. Remember that this is the birth of *your* baby and not your doctor's!

Questions to ask when choosing a doctor or midwife

When discussing your needs with the doctor or midwife choose a time when they are not in a rush. The last appointment of the day is often an ideal time as there are no other women waiting to be seen. Try to avoid making your questions seem like an interrogation. These people will be happy to give you information if you ask your questions in a relaxed, friendly manner.

- Are you in a solo practice or a partnership? Who are your partners and do you all have the same approach to the way you practise? Can I make an appointment to meet your partner(s)?
- Are you available at all times, or do you take turns to be on call during weekends?
- Do you have any plans for holidays at the time my baby is due, and who will care for me if you are away?
- What are your charges for pregnancy care, the birth and postnatal follow up? How much will I be reimbursed from Medicare?
- If I need an anaesthetic or the baby needs paediatric care, whom do you usually recommend?
- What pregnancy tests do you suggest I consider? Will you be comfortable if I choose not to have some tests, such as routine ultrasound or tests for fetal abnormalities?
- What are your preferences for management of the labour, including drugs for pain relief and positions for the birth itself? Have you ever delivered a baby with the mother squatting or kneeling on the floor? How often do you give the mother an episiotomy? How often do you use forceps?
- Will you be comfortable if I choose to have extra support people with me during the labour and birth?
- What childbirth preparation do you recommend? Where can I attend pre-natal classes?

It is useful to take your partner along on the initial visit to the doctor or midwife, as they will be sharing in the care of the pregnant mother and it is helpful for them to know each other well. Have your partner present at visits when decisions need to be made about particular aspects of pregnancy care, such as what tests to have done, or when options for birth are under discussion. An extra viewpoint and the additional support a partner provides helps the decision-making process.

3

Choosing support people

A woman labours more easily if she is supported by a select group who understand labour, know the mother well and can provide calm reassurance and privacy. Choosing the right people to be with you at this time needs careful thought and consideration. Most people love to attend a birth and are delighted to be involved, but the invitation list must be drawn up by the mother herself, if she is to feel truly comfortable with those present.

These days it is quite acceptable for the baby's father to attend the birth. While this is a radical and welcome change from his traditional role, attitudes have swung so heavily in his favour that now his presence is almost expected, and this has placed many men in a position where they feel obliged to attend, even when they would rather not. Most men enjoy the close involvement of helping at a birth and the thrill of seeing their baby born. The early contact with the baby is very beneficial and helps form close bonds between the father and his child. However, some men don't wish to be present during the labour and would prefer to limit their involvement to the time immediately after the birth of the baby. Some mothers find that the presence of the father is inhibiting during labour and that they labour more effectively if supported by other women.

It is also quite acceptable to go through birth without involving the father of the baby at all. If this approach feels right for you, do make sure that you have some other source of close support for the pregnancy, birth and the post-partum period. Good friends or empathetic family members can assist in this way and you should not hesitate to invite appropriate people to help.

The role of the support people

Support people can give the mother in labour many things: physical comfort, emotional support, reassurance, guidance, advocacy and privacy. Mothers' needs vary, from woman to woman, and also within each labour, so support people have to be alert to the changing nature and pace of labour and what is needed by the mother at any particular time.

A woman in labour needs companionship, and having close contact with supportive people has been shown to shorten the length of labour and reduce the pain. Feeling alone or being left unattended, particularly if the woman is labouring in a strange and potentially frightening environment, can make labour slower and more difficult. It was the recognition of this fact that finally opened the door for the father's presence, so that the labouring mother had the support of someone familiar in the hospital setting.

The traditional setting for birth had the mother surrounded by the other women of her group or tribe together with the midwife, or a person experienced in birthing matters. As births in western cultures were moved from the home setting to that of a hospital, these traditional supporters were excluded from the labour room, often leaving the mother alone during her labour. There were many good reasons for the presence of the support people in the traditional setting: the mother was reassured by other experienced women that labour and birth were accepted and understood as normal events in a woman's life, the baby was born into a circle of caring women and the bonding process that occurred between the baby and those present ensured that the baby would have a number of potential substitutes should the mother be unable to nurture it herself through death or illness.

Today, a woman still needs to feel surrounded by reassurance, love and acceptance and this can best be provided by those who have experienced birth themselves. In our society, extended family support is almost non-existent, yet if a mother can 'share' her baby with others who have formed close attachments to the baby at the birth, it gives her some relief from constant mothering. Birth has become more mysterious since it has occurred in hospital away from the normal daily activities of a woman's life, so extension of the birthing circle to include other women as support people can have an educative role in the community and help put birth back into its rightful place.

An extra person can help the father to enjoy the event more by providing him with emotional support and reassurance during the labour. Many men feel very uncomfortable in a hospital as it is just as unfamiliar for them, and staff sometimes expect the man to be the 'go-between' for the labouring woman and her attendants. In addition, it can be traumatic to watch a loved one go through apparent pain and discomfort for perhaps hours on end. If the support person is experienced in birth matters, her confidence and understanding can enhance the birth for both parents, and any reduction in anxiety will help remove barriers to a fast and less painful birth.

A further advantage of support people for women having babies in a hospital is that their presence gives the mother more 'say' in how she labours and gives birth. A support person can become the mother's spokesperson, and act as an intermediary between the staff and the mother to ensure that her wishes are carried out. The aim in this case is not to be an adversary, but to help provide a protected environment so that the mother can get on with her labour in peace while her supporters ensure that her needs are met.

How do you choose a support person?

It is not always easy to decide who would be the best people to have with you in labour because it is impossible to anticipate how the labour will go and what your needs will be during that time. Some women, having asked two or three people to accompany them in labour, find that they want to be by themselves and crave privacy. Others, feeling that the event should be a private affair between themselves and their partner, find that because the labour is long, a spare pair of hands would be very useful. It is probably best to adopt a flexible approach, and make it clear that support people may or may not be called to assist when the time comes.

When deciding whom to invite, some of the following points should be considered:

- How available is the person? Will they be away or at work and unable to get the time off when you need them?
- What experience do they have of birth? Are they open-minded and positive or anxious and fearful of birth themselves?
- If you are considering another mother, what were her births like? Did she labour well or did she have complications that may make her anxious when she is helping you?
- Can you feel free and uninhibited with this person? For example, would you be comfortable naked in their presence, should the need arise?
- Could you easily ask this person to leave if you find that you would prefer them to go at some time during labour?
- Would you like this person to be emotionally attached to your baby after the birth? Would they be willing to be supportive and maintain contact afterwards too?

Organising your 'team'

Once you have chosen those people who will help you during the labour and birth, it is important to spend time together talking over the plans for the birth, what everybody's role will be, and sorting out expectations. It is important that everyone feels comfortable together and that communication is open and honest.

The practical assistance that you might need should also be discussed. To help your supporters prepare well, invite them to attend your pre-natal classes so that you are all prepared in the same way for the events of the birth. Check with your childbirth educator before arriving at the class with your 'team'. Most educators will welcome their participation, and knowing that they are coming can help foster their inclusion in the class group.

Decide on an action plan for the beginning of labour. It is often best if the support people come to your house early in labour so that you can all travel together to the hospital when you feel ready to go.

For further details on how support people can be of practical assistance, have them read the chapter on labour support.

Some further considerations

When you are in the hospital, there will be midwives available who can provide extra assistance and support. This is the normal role of the midwife and she will welcome the chance to be part of your 'team'. Sometimes, however, staffing shortages or a busy labour ward dictate that the midwives can't spend as much time with you as you would like, and this is where having your own support people on hand can ensure the practical help you need.

Some mothers prefer to engage a private midwife or childbirth educator to provide more professional support during labour and birth. These people have extensive experience of birth and can often judge when it is the best time to go to the hospital. This allows the mother to stay at home in her own environment for longer and minimises the length of time necessary in hospital.

Hospitals can be busy places, especially if they are teaching hospitals for midwives or medical students. The private event you had planned for youself and your partner can become very public if students or other staff invade your cosy birthplace. You have the right to ask these extras to leave if they are a disturbance. Sometimes an extra support person can act as a filter between both of you and the extra staff.

One of the greatest disturbances for a woman in labour is having too many people disrupting the flow of labour in some way. When choosing support people to help you in labour, keep this in mind. There will be a number of midwives, other staff and perhaps students present from time to time during the labour, and if you have more than two support people of your own quite a crowd could form! More people mean more noise, and the potential for more distraction. As the crowd grows, your feeling of privacy diminishes and this can slow labour down. If you sense that there are too many people present, you can always ask some of them to leave or you can escape to a small quiet place for a time such as the toilet or shower.

It is probably better to have one or two support people with you for the duration of the labour rather than a team of people who take it in turns to come and go. When you have constant support, your needs can be better understood and the rhythm of labour is not interrupted. If one person has just the right knack of rubbing your back, then you will want that person to stay with you, rather than have to explain to a succession of people just where you want the pressure etc. Be wary of 'visitors' who come up to the hospital to see how things are going and invite themselves into the labour room. These visits are more social events, and it can be hard to overcome your natural tendency to 'socialise' to concentrate on the labour. If you do have visitors, ask your main support person to see them outside and give them a progress report. Try not to let their presence or their expectations disrupt the flow of labour.

4

Pre-natal preparation

Attending pre-natal classes can be of great value during your pregnancy. Although no one can teach you how to have a baby, the contact with other parents and the information about the labour process, pregnancy and parenting and your choices and options can be very useful.

Some years ago, the primary aim of pre-natal classes was to teach women patterned behaviour that would help them achieve a painless childbirth. Many parents have heard of the 'breathing' that formed one of the cornerstones of this kind of teaching. We now know that teaching women these distraction techniques, especially breathing patterns, can be unhelpful and at times dangerous. To labour easily, a woman needs to be free of any learned behaviour so that she can readily tune in to her body and be ready to respond to its needs as necessary. The process of labour is powerful and at times overwhelming, and trying to avoid the sensations by using an intellectual, learned pattern of behaviour can cause anxiety in the mother, especially if it is not effective, with a consequent slowing of labour and increase in the level of pain. The baby is also at greater risk of distress if the mother needs medical assistance or drugs as a result of the slow, painful labour.

Once these potential problems were recognised, pre-natal teaching swung away from instruction in 'methods' for childbirth and concentrated more on a physiologic approach, with an emphasis on helping women gain confidence in their own abilities to give birth. In addition, more time is now spent on explaining choices and options in care and management, all of which help a mother to labour in her own way. The social aspect of classes, the need to be with other pregnant women and their partners to exchange views, attitudes and problems now has greater emphasis, especially with our more isolated family units in the community.

Pre-natal classes

There are many different types of pre-natal classes available, and it is worth asking your friends and professional advisers for information on what is available near you. You will probably want to talk to the educator who is running the classes to find out what they will cover and some details about their format.

Classes can be structured in various ways:

- informal classes run on an 'open door' principle. Mothers can attend a group whenever they feel able. This is convenient for some, but tends to lead to lack of continuity in the group and in the information being offered. They are often run in conjunction with outpatient clinic appointments, and may be available only for the mothers. Booking is probably not necessary.
- lecture style classes, where an audience is addressed by a number of speakers on a set series of topics, with time for questions at the end. This format is popular with hospitals where a large number of parents request classes. The problem with this approach is that there is very little time for individual questions or attention. These classes are usually offered in the evening so that both parents can attend and booking is necessary.
- exercise classes, where the emphasis is on stretching, getting fit and general toning up. These classes are usually run by a physiotherapist, and are generally for women only, during the day. Booking is essential.
- combined exercise, mothercraft and labour classes. These are usually presented by a small team who each take part of the class. For example, the first hour may be an exercise session, followed by an hour of labour discussion or babycare or parenting information. The format varies according to the team and the amount of time available. These classes are designed for both parents so usually take place at night and the group size is kept small to encourage participation. Booking is essential.
- integrated classes, where the full class series is taught by one childbirth educator who covers all the information on pregnancy, labour and parenting as a continuum. Class sizes are usually small, both parents are expected to attend, and support people are welcome. These classes offer the greatest opportunity for individual needs to be met within the group and for the information to be linked together in a smooth related format. Booking is essential.

There are a number of other class formats that may also be available, either separately or as part of one of the class series described above.

Pregnancy classes (sometimes called 'early bird classes'): these are scheduled for parents in the early part of pregnancy, preferably about 12–16 weeks. They give the opportunity to gain information about the pregnancy, self-help ideas for making this time more comfortable, background details about tests, and consumer information about choosing doctors, hospitals etc. Some integrated classes are arranged so that the first classes are done in this early stage of pregnancy, with the same group attending birth classes closer to the birth date.

Refresher classes: these are designed for parents who already have a child and who want to 'refresh' themselves about the birth process and labour management techniques. The format may include two or more classes or may be offered as private lessons by an independent educator. The content is often less structured than classes for first-time parents, and time is usually allocated for questions and discussion according to the needs of the parents.

Parenting classes: most pre-natal classes include some information on parenting issues and babycare. Sometimes this is given in a separate session just for the mothers, or it may be included towards the end of the class series following the information on the birth. Most parenting classes today include the father in recognition of his greater role in raising the children. Some educators offer separate parenting classes either as one or two classes in the middle or end of the pregnancy, or sometimes as a series following the birth, over a number of weeks. These post-natal parenting groups can be very helpful and provide much practical assistance and support particularly for first-time parents.

Sibling classes: these are designed to help children prepare for the arrival of a new brother or sister. They are often provided as an offshoot from refresher classes, and their availability tends to be variable, according to need.

When you are making your decision about which classes to attend, asking the following questions will give you the answers you need to make an informed choice.

- At what stage in the pregnancy do I begin the classes?
- Where and when are the classes held?
- Can my partner and my support people attend the group?
- How large are the class groups?

- Who leads the classes: a single educator, or is there a team approach?
- How much do the classes cost? Are rebates available from any source?
- Is there any post-natal follow up, or class reunion?
- What do the classes cover? Are books and other literature available to borrow? Do we see videos?
- What handouts are given to class participants?
- Is the educator available for consultation by phone or in person between the classes if I need special help or want to ask a specific question?
- Will we see the labour ward as part of the class or should I arrange this separately?
- What is the overall philosophy of the classes: do they encourage me to use my own resources and make my own decisions or do they emphasise preparing me for what the hospital will expect me to do during labour?

Your childbirth educator

The people who conduct pre-natal classes are called childbirth educators. Some may have other talents as well and work in different areas at other times, such as midwifery, physiotherapy or another field. Childbirth educators should have special skills that enable them to teach adults effectively in a small group setting, as well as having a broad knowledge of pregnancy, birth and post-natal subjects. Most have done special training and continue to update their knowledge and skills through reading and by attending seminars and workshops.

Many educators have experienced birth themselves, but this is not essential, just as it is not required for other professionals to have had personal experiences similar to the people they are helping. Given that birth is infinitely variable, it is unlikely that your educator will have been in a situation that will mirror your own, when the time comes. Educators know this, and keep their own birth stories out of classes. They will, however, have a good knowledge of birth from attending labours, and they have a commitment and enthusiasm for birth that you will find reassuring.

It is not necessary to have a referral from your doctor before going to classes. It is useful to tell the doctor that you are attending classes with your partner as this will let him or her know that you are interested in finding out about birth and that you will probably have questions to ask. If your doctor is wary of your going to a pre-natal class, ask why she holds these views. Some doctors prefer their patients to be uninformed as this makes it easier to manage the labour according to the doctor's wishes.

5

Making pregnancy comfortable

Although pregnancy is a normal condition for a woman, there are some side effects that can be annoying and there are things you can do to make the pregnancy easier.

Firstly, assume that all is well. Don't be alarmed by the odd aches and pains that occur and the strange sensations that you feel from time to time. These are all probably normal, although not all women suffer from them and you may feel that your symptoms are unique. Talking to other women will reassure you that others have similar reminders of pregnancy to contend with, but if you are truly concerned, speak to your midwife or doctor (phone, don't wait for your next visit) or ask your childbirth educator.

Secondly, ignore negative comments about your age, the number of children you already have and any superstitious remarks offered by others. The notion that age is a factor influencing the outcome of your pregnancy is particularly unhelpful. Many women today are choosing to have babies later in life, and they are at no particular increased risk as long as their general health is good and they take the usual care of themselves through the pregnancy. Additional pregnancy tests for malformations in the baby are often stressed as important for the older mother, but these need to be considered carefully, as they carry risks themselves which may be greater than the chance of the baby having a problem. This issue is discussed further on page 28.

Accepting your pregnancy

While your body will react and adapt to the growing baby in its own way, you don't need to assume that many of your usual activities are now 'out of bounds'. A pregnant woman can do most things as long as some common sense is applied to avoid undue fatigue or strain. As the baby grows your capacity for exercise will gradually decrease, but this does not mean you have to become a lounge lizard—just modify your activities to a level that remains comfortable. Indeed, some women benefit from beginning some gentle exercise at this time, especially walking or swimming, which can help you to feel good while giving your body the gentle exercise it still needs.

You will probably notice emotional swings and mood changes over the months of pregnancy too. In the first few months many women need time to come to terms with being pregnant, even if the baby is planned and very much wanted. These feelings of ambivalence can be surprising, and some mothers have said that they felt they needed the full nine months to really get used to the idea of becoming a parent. The mood swings and increased intensity of emotional reactions can catch some mothers by surprise as well, and bewilder even the most tolerant partner. Although caused by the pregnancy hormones, it is not enough to dismiss these reactions as 'hormonal'. A woman needs some reassurance and understanding as well as calm tolerance and acceptance. Being able to talk about these needs is often a great help.

Changing body shape and a rearrangement of one's body image is necessary during pregnancy. Some women adore the growing belly while others find the swollen tummy difficult to accommodate, both physically and emotionally. Pregnancy forces a woman to reconsider how she feels about her sexuality and her partner also needs to consider her new role as a mother as well as a lover. Sex itself needs some adaptation, which can be enjoyable for the open and adventurous but threatening for couples whose relationship is stressed in any way. Again, talking about these issues with each other, as well as with sympathetic friends or counsellors can often do much to ease any strains.

The decision about when to leave work also needs to be considered. You may be able to work through most of your pregnancy, but it will depend on the job you have and the physical and emotional stresses it imposes. If you notice an increasing need for sleep, a lowered tolerance for dealing with other people's problems, daydreaming and a lack of concentration on your work, then these may be signals that you are ready for a rest in preparation for the birth and later parenting. Leaving work will mean adjusting to one income instead of two, and this can impose pressures to stay at work as long as possible. Since it is known that babies grow better when the mother avoids heavy physical work in the last months of pregnancy, this also needs to be weighed up against the need for additional income. Finding the right decision for you will need discussion with your partner and careful consideration of your position and physical health.

Your life together will never be the same once the baby arrives, and the changes wrought by the pregnancy will help you prepare for this. Already you are probably more aware than ever before of what you are eating, your activities, your living conditions, social circle, support networks and attitudes to becoming parents.

When you are scrutinising your lifestyle in preparation for further changes, remember that a baby's basic needs are for love, acceptance and nurturing. There is no need to set yourself impossible standards for housing the baby—your child will need you as a person more than it needs pretty wallpaper or a special room. You can transport a baby just as easily in a sling or backpack as in an elaborate pram that sets you back financially for months. Relatives and friends would probably be delighted to give or lend you baby equipment they don't need at the present time and this will save you money and reduce the financial burden of raising your family.

Similarly, you may be able to make do with your current accommodation by having the baby share your room initially. When the child is more mobile and needs extra space for play it may be time to move to a larger house. Many families try to build an extra room or move to a larger home while the pregnancy is in progress. This can place an added strain on the mother, both physically and emotionally, and this should be considered. Many women are driven by a strong nesting urge, but coping with renovations, disrupted households and physical difficulties can be a high price to pay.

Medical care in pregnancy

Most women have regular checks during their pregnancies, beginning with monthly visits to their midwife or doctor, then fortnightly and weekly visits as the pregnancy nears its end. There are a number of standard assessments made at these visits and there are additional tests that can be carried out if circumstances suggest they would be advisable.

An initial test is done to confirm the pregnancy. Following this, blood tests to determine blood group, rubella protection level, iron levels, and exposure to sexually transmitted diseases are carried out. Additional blood tests may be ordered if the mother or baby show signs of poor health.

Around 16 weeks further diagnostic tests may be suggested: ultrasound to check the baby's size and potential birth date, amniocentesis to check for fetal abnormalities, and further blood tests to check on the baby's well-being. It is not necessary to have all of these tests done, even though you may be strongly advised to go ahead. Before you make the decision to submit to the test, find out as much as you can about its risks and benefits: *Preparing for Birth* (see 'Further Reading' for details) or a comprehensive book on pregnancy will give you the information you need.

Whenever you are offered medical tests in your pregnancy (or at any other time), there are a number of questions you should ask.

• What is the test? How it is it done? What will the results tell us?
• How will having the test done alter the current or proposed treatment?
• What side effects could I experience? Are there any risks associated with the test?
• Are there alternative tests available?
• What happens if I choose not to have the test?

You should also ask these questions if you are being prescribed drugs of any kind. Just substitute the word 'drug' for 'test' in the above questions.

If you find it difficult to ask the doctor or midwife these kinds of questions, you may be helped by one or more of the following ideas.

• Write the question down and have it in your hand when you make your visit. Try not to leave it in your bag by mistake!
• Ask your questions when you are sitting opposite the doctor or midwife after the examination has been completed. Don't try to ask questions when you are lying down looking up at the doctor. This is a very vulnerable position to be in and will sap your confidence.
• Take a support person with you to the consultation. The importance of the situation to you will be underlined and you will have more time spent with you. A male supporter will probably be useful if you are dealing with a male doctor.

Ask for time to consider the answers you have been given before agreeing to any course of action. Avoid being bulldozed into the suggested treatment without having time to think about your options. You may want to consult your support person and you may also want to consider getting a second medical opinion. Very few situations are so urgent that instant medical decisions need to be made, and you may find that sleeping on it, and considering your options away from the shock or stress of discovering that there is a problem, helps you to make a good decision.

Obtaining a second medical opinion

It might help to get a second medical opinion from someone who can review the situation from a fresh viewpoint. Doctors who work in partnership often have similar views and methods, so it might be better to see a doctor from a different practice, or even the next town. In rural areas there are often fewer doctors from whom to choose and the way they approach any problem may be very similar. If the issue is very important to you (for example, where your doctor is suggesting a caesarian rather than a vaginal birth for a breech baby and you would prefer to try for a normal birth) it might be worth travelling even as far as a major centre or capital city where the range of opinions is wider and there are more doctors with innovative ideas.

If you want to arrange a second opinion, the first step is to find a suitable doctor who will see you quickly and consider your case. You could seek suggestions from your childbirth educator or midwife about possible doctors you could see. These people are in a good position to know of alternative ways of managing a problem and may have had other clients who have been in similar situations. Alternatively, you may be able to locate other women who could pass on information from a similar experience.

Next, phone for an appointment with the second doctor and explain to the secretary that you are seeking a second opinion and that you want an appointment that will allow enough time for discussion, perhaps the last appointment for the day. When this is settled, you will have to visit your general practitioner and obtain a letter of referral to the second doctor. This should present no problems.

While you are awaiting the appointment, you should become as informed as you can about your problem so you have some idea of what alternatives may be suggested. It is very hard to know what questions to ask unless you have some knowledge of your own condition. Again, your childbirth educator or midwife should be able to suggest useful reading matter.

Once you have seen the second doctor, and heard his suggestions and advice, you will have to decide what course of action you wish to take. You may decide to stay with your first choice of doctor, and either carry on as planned or ask him to modify his approach. Alternatively you may decide to change doctors so that a fresh start is made with a different management plan.

Changing doctors

If you decide at any time that the care you are receiving from your doctor is not what you are looking for, you are quite free to change doctors. Many women find this hard to do during pregnancy, because it is hard to acknowledge that the care offered is not what you want or need and it takes an effort to change to someone who will give you what you want. Pregnant women are very vulnerable emotionally and psychologically and need to feel protected and nurtured by health professionals who will listen and make an effort to provide for the mother's individual needs. During pregnancy, a woman usually has to undergo several intimate pelvic examinations, and you know that during the labour you will also be exposed physically and emotionally. It is easier to accept these situations if you have a good relationship with the midwife or doctor and feel comfortable with their presence. Being able to talk freely with someone who listens and takes heed is an important part of this process.

If, even right near the end of your pregnancy, you feel that these conditions are not developing, then it may be better to change to someone who is more suited to you. Labour will be faster and easier if you know you can trust those taking care of you, so changing doctors may have great benefits in the long run.

It is quite easy to change doctors, and patients do this all the time in other areas of medicine. It is wise to have a consultation with the new doctor to make sure that they are going to be suitable—you can use the guidelines for seeking a second opinion to help you in this process. After the consultation, if you decide that you want to change to this new doctor or midwife, contact the first doctor or midwife and explain to the secretary that you have decided to go elsewhere and request that your medical records be sent to the new doctor or midwife. This is quite ethical and is simply done. It would also be courteous to see or write to the former carer, explain your reasons for changing and thank them for their help so far.

Don't feel embarrassed by this procedure. Doctors are quite used to women switching doctors during pregnancy, and there is a chance that they will be quite glad for you to move if your requests are going to be hard to meet. Personality clashes are quite common in everyday life, so it is to be expected that these can occur in the doctor/patient relationship too.

One additional benefit of changing your doctor, apart from making your own birth easier and more enjoyable, is that such consumer pressure is powerful in encouraging midwives and doctors to reassess their methods of treatment. If enough women exercise their right to change doctors then the effects will certainly be noticed, and those professionals who provide the best service and the most flexibility will benefit. Many of the changes that have occurred in the area of childbirth have been brought about because women asked and even insisted on doing something different, not because a doctor or midwife thought it would be nice to try another way of managing birth. You are in a powerful position to influence change, not only in terms of your own baby and body, but also in helping make those responsible for maternity care more sensitive and responsive.

Developing support networks

The months of pregnancy are a good time to begin developing a network of contacts who can provide you with social outlets, physical help, and emotional and psychological support both during your pregnancy and after the baby is born. Your partner will probably be your major source of support but you will also need the company and contact of other women who also have, or are expecting, babies. There are lots of things about being a mother that men may have trouble understanding, and it is very reassuring to be able to compare notes with other mothers and learn from each other's experiences.

Men also need a support network, perhaps drawn from amongst friends or workmates. Being a father is a new experience with its own set of worries, pleasures and questions. This need of new fathers for support is not well recognised in our community, yet if the men felt more comfortable and happy in their role as fathers they could often provide better support for the mother of their child.

Pregnancy and birth are unique and special but are experiences with many similarities for all women. It is comforting to know that what you are feeling has been felt by others and that the new sensations and emotional upheavals that occur have been shared by other women over the generations. Once you begin talking to other women about having babies, the common features of pregnancy and birth can be better understood and the new mother can be reassured that all is well. This kind of sharing can develop only amongst women. There are a number of ways that you can develop a circle of supportive friends.

Overcome your shyness and speak to everyone you see or meet

who is pregnant. You will see pregnant women in the street, going to work, in shops where you are both buying baby needs, waiting to see the doctor, at the hospital clinic and in lots of other places. You have probably not noticed how many pregnant women there are until now! You all have at least one thing in common, a growing baby inside, and talking to other expectant mothers is usually welcomed. Pluck up your courage and start a conversation!

The other people at your pre-natal class probably live in your area and would welcome the chance to develop some social contacts. You will all have babies of about the same age, and this is particularly helpful later when you can all compare notes on your mothering experiences and your babies' development. Some childbirth educators provide a list of names and addresses for the participants in their groups, but you could easily do this yourself if it is not provided, by swapping names and phone numbers during the refreshment break at the class.

Join an exercise group, particularly if it is aimed at pregnant women. You will have lots of fun and the companionship of other women is an important element of these groups.

Attend the meetings of any parenting groups that are available in your area. The Nursing Mothers Association of Australia, for example, hold meetings for breastfeeding mothers, and they particularly welcome pregnant women at these groups. There are Childbirth and Parenting groups in many towns and cities. The Infant Welfare Centre or Community Health Centre will have a list of other groups in your area that might also be of interest. Playgroups too provide a great opportunity for meeting other families. Although designed primarily to meet children's needs for group play, a playgroup is also a group meeting place for parents, since the child must be accompanied by an adult. Enquire about babysitting groups or clubs, and child care centres in your area. These all cater for parents so could help you to make valuable contacts.

Suggestions for support people of the pregnant woman

Your basic role as a support person during her pregnancy will be to protect her from undue worries, encourage and reassure her in moments of doubt, provide physical comfort and offer a listening ear when needed. You may need some support yourself during this time, so having a team of support people is a good idea, to spread the load and to allow you all more enjoyment during this exciting time.

Below are some some practical ideas that may be appreciated by the pregnant mother.

- Spend time with her regularly to share thoughts and feelings about the pregnancy, the birth and the prospect of parenthood. Putting some time aside for this purpose not only acknowledges her need to share feelings, but is a tangible measure of your involvement and concern. You will also feel supported and involved.

- Ease her aches and pains as much as you can. Some massage, hot packs, extra pillows in bed, lumbar support in the car and accommodating her changed eating patterns will be much appreciated. Don't be unduly alarmed by physical symptoms as most women's bodies complain as they adjust to the growing baby and most of the symptoms are temporary in nature. She will need to avoid heavy lifting and be aware that as her tummy grows her centre of balance will change—she may not be safe up a ladder painting any more!

- Although physical symptoms are often nothing more than minor annoyances, don't dismiss them or under-rate the discomfort they may cause. If she says she is worried about a particular problem, encourage her to speak to the doctor, midwife or childbirth educator about it. She doesn't have to wait until the next visit, as these people are available by phone. Should she notice any bleeding, contractions or leaking membranes (especially before 37 weeks of pregnancy) then take her to the doctor or hospital straight away. Bleeding (not spotting, which is normal) could indicate problems with the placenta, and contractions or leaking membranes could mean the start of labour. If this happens before 37 weeks it may be possible to stop the labour proceeding and so help to avoid problems associated with prematurity for the baby.

- Encourage her to keep as physically active as she can, without overdoing the exercise or straining herself unnecessarily. Listen to her wishes about staying at work or leaving to get more rest. Although the extra income may be needed, it will have to weighed up against the potential for undermining the health of the mother and baby if she stays on at work when it is beyond her capacity to cope with it.

- Humour her changes in mood and personality. The emotional see-saws are bewildering and surprising for her too: you can both laugh about it in the future!

- Attend the pre-natal visits to the doctor or midwife as often as you can, both to give her support and to have your own questions answered. You will feel more involved and she will get more attention if there are two of you.

- Go to the classes with her. You will be surprised how much you learn and you will feel more confident when you are better prepared for the birth. All the birth support people should go to the birth classes so that you all learn to work as a team and you are all in the picture about possible events and practical measures you can offer to ease her pain. There is more on this in a later chapter.

• Most of all, communicate with her. Share your feelings, work together on problems and develop new understandings in your relationship with her. A pregnant woman needs good communication not only with her partner, but with her women friends, relatives and caregivers too. These developments will also form a good basis for support in the post-natal period, which is often a time of great stress for new parents.

The better you get to know the mother now, the more you will be able to offer later. It may seem like a one-way street at times, with much giving on your behalf and little in return. The benefits for you will come later, when she can support you in turn and give you the benefit of her new insights. In today's society, especially with its isolated nuclear families, we need better support networks throughout the community, to foster well-being and give life a sense of purpose. This is a good time to start reaching out to each other in a new way that will give immediate and tangible results. There is nothing like the arrival of a new baby to create and strengthen bonds amongst people. Enjoy and discover for yourself!

6

Preparing your other children

If you have other children, preparing them for the arrival of a brother or sister will help you feel more at ease during the pregnancy and labour. How much you involve them in the preparations for the birth, and what arrangements you make for them at the time of the labour will depend on their ages and their level of interest. Young children are often quite fascinated by the baby growing in their mother's tummy and they can be very curious about how the baby will be born.

Older children also like to be involved. They can enjoy helping to prepare a place for the new baby and doing small tasks for you. The following suggestions may be useful as you prepare your children.

Tell the children about the coming baby when you feel it is appropriate. Siblings need time to adjust to the news and make their own preparations for the new baby, so allow them several months. Young children have no real understanding of time and can become tired of waiting if you tell them too soon: perhaps the best time is when the baby starts to make its presence felt by kicking inside your tummy. Older children may need to know earlier than this so they understand the side effects of pregnancy that may be making an impact on the family (for example, fatigue, morning sickness etc).

Answer questions as honestly as you can and use books, pictures or videos to back up your information. Children take these sexual topics in their stride much more easily than adults and can be surprisingly matter-of-fact if you are open and allow free discussion. Using the correct names for body parts and emphasising the positive and exciting aspects of the event will help them develop a good attitude towards birth that will pay dividends in their later lives. Your childbirth educator or local librarian can help you locate books for children on birth topics.

If the children are interested, take them on some of your prenatal visits to the doctor. They can listen to the baby's heart, feel the baby in your tummy and begin to understand what will happen during the birth. Meeting the doctor is also important if you plan to have the other children at the birth.

Many children like to be involved in making a place ready for the baby, choosing clothes and toys and so on. This will help them to accept a new member of the family and to understand the preparations that were made for their own arrival. Explaining how you readied everything for their birth is a great way of acknowledging how special they are as a person, and will help build a child's self-esteem. If you have some photos of them as babies, or even pictures taken at the birth, they will be fascinated and will probably want to see them over and over again.

Some women want to involve the other siblings at the birth and some children express a strong desire to be there. For you to labour easily, you will need to feel uninhibited and free to express your feelings, so you will need to consider whether having your other children present will make this difficult. As it is always hard to anticipate how the birth will go, and how you will feel at the time, it is probably wise to keep your options open right up till the baby is born. Make suitable arrangements for care of the children at the birth so they can be taken out should you or they be disturbed by what is happening.

Young children (under 4 years) don't always have enough language to express what they are feeling, although they usually can understand much more than you think. They can often cope quite well with birth, provided that they are not expected to behave in an unnatural way (being alert at 3.00 a.m. or amusing themselves for hours in an unfamiliar hospital, for example) and have a constant caregiver who will attend to their needs at all times. One of the members of your support team should be happy to take on this responsibility.

Older children will also need someone to take care of them during the birth. Giving each child a specific job, such as bringing drinks of water or wiping their mother's forehead, can help them participate positively. Teenage children, particularly girls, sometimes find birth too confronting, as they struggle to establish their own sexuality. You will know your own children and what they are capable of gaining from participation in the birth. The important thing is not to force them to join in and not to underestimate the effect they may have on you when you are in labour.

If your children are going to be at the birth, then you will need to spend time explaining what they will see and hear. Videos may be useful, but choose them with care and make sure you have viewed them first before you show them to your children. Your childbirth educator may be able to lend you a video or a set of photos that could be used as a substitute. Photos have the advantage of being able to be discussed individually at you and your children's pace.

Make some contingency plans for the birth should you decide at the last moment that you don't want the children present. Having a babysitter on call, a neighbour available or a live-in relative will allow you to reassess the situation at any time. You will probably want to stay at home as long as possible whether you are taking your children to hospital with you or not, to avoid disrupting the family too much. Have a 'hospital' bag packed for your children too, with toys, books, food snacks and a drink to help keep them happy while you are labouring.

If you are planning a homebirth, then preparing the children will be essential. It is still a good idea to have a helper for the children, so that you can labour in peace. If the labour is mainly in the day, then let the children carry on as usual: you will probably find they appear and disappear to suit the level of involvement they wish to have. If it is at night, then they will need to be woken in time for the birth according to how much time they need to wake properly. A sleepy child who wakes badly may be better left to sleep. Thrusting a half-awake child into a birth room could leave the impression of a nightmare!

Choose carers for your children who know them well, whether you are having the children with you at the birth or not. You will labour with an easier mind if you know that your children are being cared for by someone who understands them and can keep them happy for many hours if needed. Immediate phone contact after the birth, and bringing the children to see you just after the birth to meet the new baby are good alternatives for most families who don't want the other children present for the birth itself.

After the birth

Consider how long you want to stay in hospital after the baby is born. You may miss your other children, but may also be enjoying the break from household routine. Going home early will help avoid separation traumas especially for children under 3 years old. If you can arrange suitable help at home early discharge is often the best plan, provided that you are allowed to spend time with the baby and do no household tasks or cooking for some days. If this help cannot be arranged, then you may be better off in hospital.

Be prepared for some regression and adverse behaviour in your other children in the first few months after the new baby's arrival. It is inevitable that other children will feel displaced to some degree, and with the focus of attention firmly on the new baby, they often feel left out and rejected. Try to keep the children's routine as normal as possible and avoid always asking them to make way for the baby. You could try to spend more time with the baby in the evening (bathing, playing, etc) when the other children are asleep, so that you can give attention to your other children during the day. Your partner could spend more time with the children in the first few months and this will help prevent your other children from feeling displaced by the baby.

Many mothers worry about being able to love the new baby as much as their other children. It is amazing how love can expand to encompass all, and you may be surprised at the capacity you have to give of yourself to so many people! A baby has magical ways of engendering love in others, and even if it does not come immediately at birth, love grows and the new baby will take its place with your other children in your affections.

7

Birth plans

When you are in labour, you will not always be able to communicate your wishes and decisions easily to those looking after you, because you will be concentrating on what is happening in your body and discussion with others can be impossible, even undesirable.

A birth plan is a statement about how you would like your birth to be managed. By indicating on a birth plan your wishes and feelings about the way you want the birth to go, you will lay the groundwork for good communication during labour and birth and make it much easier for those with you to ensure that your wishes are respected.

It is important however to keep an open mind as labour progresses, because you may wish to change your mind, or circumstances may mean that your preferred options can no longer be considered. A birth plan should never lock you into one plan of management; it should be designed to indicate your preferences overall. For example, you may have decided that you would prefer not to have an episiotomy (a cut in the vaginal wall to enlarge the opening for birth) as a routine measure. If however, the baby shows signs of distress, you may welcome an episiotomy as a way of speeding up the birth in second stage so that the baby can be helped sooner. This kind of decision must be made at the time, and so you need to have flexibility in your approach.

A list of suggested inclusions on a birth plan appears in *Preparing for Birth*. These are intended only as a guide, and you can include anything else that you feel is important. Remember to consider your choices for the pregnancy and the post-natal period, both of which take much longer than the labour!

Before you can compile a useful birth plan, you will need to have access to information about your various options. Attending pre-natal classes will give you an opportunity to find out about alternatives in pregnancy and labour care, and the hospital staff can tell you about routines and staff preferences on your labour ward tour.

Once you have formulated your birth plan, the next step is to discuss it with the people who will be with you during labour so that everyone is clear about your wishes. There are three people who need to be fully informed.

First you should tell your support person(s). It is essential for those who will support you during labour to know what you want to do, to understand their role and to know what they expect of each other. Discuss it as a group a few weeks before the birth and make sure that everyone is clear. If you wish your support people to take an advocacy role and speak to staff on your behalf, then this must be understood by your supporters and also by the staff, who often distrust support people in this role (for example 'What would they know—they are not having the baby!').

Secondly the midwife or midwives who will care for you in labour need to be informed of your plans. Talking to them in advance will help you to discover hospital policy and also help them to know you and your needs. If you arrive in labour to find an unfamiliar midwife greeting you, give her a copy of the birth plan and try to find a few minutes to enlist her help. The midwife needs to be clear about what you want as she will be relaying reports about your progress to the doctor and acting as your advocate, or spokesperson, with the doctor. The midwife will be with you for all of the labour, and if she understands what you want to do, she can make sure that your wishes are carried out. Having written instructions on your birth plan will make her job much easier, as your plan can be attached to your nursing notes so that all staff members know what you require. These notes also form clear guidelines for consent purposes and help define legal limitations on what can be done by the midwife and doctor.

Finally you must discuss your plans with your doctor. While many midwives welcome the challenge of varying ways of managing labour, there can be resistance from some doctors to varying the way in which they manage your labour and birth. The birth plan will give you a starting point for negotiation, and help you to establish their approach and methods. While it is unfair to expect that a doctor should be comfortable with new ideas immediately (for example, squatting for the birth) they should be prepared to discuss their views honestly and explain their position so that you are fully aware of their attitudes. If the doctor is unwilling to negotiate or accommodate your needs, then you may wish to get a second opinion or change doctors. Often however, with communication and goodwill on both sides a compromise position can be established and with luck, the doctor will learn some new techniques!

Keep updating your birth plan as the pregnancy progresses. Developments in your health or that of the baby may mean that you have to modify your birth plan to ensure safety. For example, if you begin labour prematurely, you may have to change your plans for a home birth to one at the hospital where specialised equipment is available should the baby need it immediately. Not all apparent complications, however, mean that you have to abandon your plans completely. For example, if the baby seems distressed during labour and electronic fetal monitoring equipment needs to be attached to chart the baby's reactions, you don't necessarily need to abandon your plans to be upright and mobile during labour. You can still sit or stand beside the bed, even with the fetal monitor attached, and being upright will reduce the possibility of further fetal distress due to lying down. Flexibility is the key in using a birth plan, with constant modifications and updates as the pregnancy and labour unfolds.

If you make several copies of your birth plan then you can keep a copy, one can be given to the doctor and another can be attached to your hospital records. It might be helpful to have your doctor sign the plan before you make the copies as this will then act as a set of instructions to the hospital staff, should he or she be unavailable to explain your wishes verbally at the beginning of labour. In most hospitals, the staff keep a list of each doctor's preferred management plan and use this as a guide for their patients when they are admitted. If you have negotiated a different management plan from the doctor's usual methods then it would be wise to have this in writing from the doctor (either in a letter of referral or a signed birth plan) so you can present it on his behalf when you book in for labour. In this way there will be no confusion, and the midwives will be clear about the changes in your particular case.

When you present your birth plan to the midwife on your arrival at the hospital, use a friendly assertive approach. Ask the midwife to assist you in achieving your goals rather than demanding that 'This is what we want!'. Everyone responds favourably to a pleasant request, but a strident demand can be met with hostility. This will create a difficult atmosphere that will not make the labour easier for anyone.

In addition, many midwives are only too willing to help you in every way, but know that this might make them unpopular with the doctors in some cases. This places them in the very difficult position of being caught in the middle between you and your doctor. If you understand this, you can be supportive of the midwife, and give her permission to act on your behalf, a position that is readily assumed by most midwives, who see *you* as their primary responsibility, not the doctor and his preferred practices. You need the midwife's support, and she needs yours. Together you can more readily achieve the birth that you desire.

Perhaps right now you are feeling that all of these suggestions are too difficult to attempt or not necessary because you have faith in your doctor or midwife and trust their judgement. The birth experience is an individual event and your experience will be shaped by many factors. You can do much to ensure that the birth goes the way you want it to, but it will take some work to think the issues through and to make the appropriate plans. You can put all your faith in the doctor and hospital staff, but they will give you an experience that matches their expectations, and not necessarily yours. You may be quite happy with this approach as it requires less effort on your part and you may be just wanting to get the baby born, rather than seeking an individual experience. Whichever way you decide to prepare for the birth, it will almost certainly turn out to be different from what you expected, and will need some reassessment after the event.

8

Your legal rights

At all times you have a right to know about any matter that affects you or your baby. You have a right to information presented in a way that you can understand, to the results of tests that may be done on you or the baby, and to participation in any decisions about treatment that are undertaken. You have a right to ask questions and receive answers.

Having asked a doctor or midwife to undertake your pregnancy care and to help at the birth of the baby, you have a 'contract' whereby you agree to allow them to treat you (with your permission) and to make decisions about your care (after you have been consulted). You agree to disclose any information they need to allow them to treat you properly and to carry out the agreed treatment to the best of your ability.

Before a doctor or midwife can give you any treatment or carry out any procedure, they have to make sure that you understand the nature of the treatment or procedure, its alternatives, its advantages and disadvantages and the expected results or side effects. Many mothers put their faith in a doctor and never question what he does, yet are surprised that there are side effects or disadvantages afterwards that they had not been told about. Just as the doctor has a responsibility to tell you what he plans to do and to get your informed consent, you have a responsibility to ask questions, to consider the alternatives and to be as fully informed as possible.

If drugs are prescribed you should check what they are, what they will do and what side effects can be expected. In return, you should inform the doctor of any drugs you are already taking, and take any medication strictly as directed. It helps to keep a record of drugs you have taken so that you know in the future what chemicals your baby has been exposed to.

You should also be given the results of any tests that you have paid for, in a written form if requested. This is also true of ultrasounds and X-rays, which are your property, as you have paid for them.

There are a number of possible medical interventions in labour that are controversial, such as electronic fetal monitoring, ultrasound, routine caesarian sections for breech babies, lying down for the birth, routine administration of oxytocin for third stage and routine rupture of membranes in labour, to mention just a few. Some people would say that any intervention in the normal process of birth is questionable unless it is clearly evident that the baby requires immediate rescue, or that the mother's life is in danger. Because these procedures are controversial, many doctors and midwives will have their own views that they will defend strenuously if questioned. It can be hard to argue against such strong views, especially when dealing with a professional person who may use language you don't understand or even emotional arguments to sway you to their point of view. If this happens, a second opinion can help you decide for yourself, and extra reading and information will be essential. If the procedure in question is a very important issue for you, remember that the doctor or midwife has to obtain your permission before they can proceed, otherwise they may be legally at fault. Once you have agreed to be their patient, they assume responsibility for your care and outcome, and this is a serious undertaking, especially if things go wrong. If you are asking them to do something that they feel is against their normal practice, then they will be unwilling to take responsibility, which is their right. You may be asked to take responsibility for the outcome, and to sign a statement to this effect, perhaps in your medical notes at the hospital.

Writing your wishes down (either as a birth plan or as a note you ask the midwife to enter in your records) not only clarifies the situation but makes it impossible for the doctor to intervene or go against your expressed wishes without risking legal liabilities. This can be a useful, although heavy-handed, technique if you are dealing with a doctor who seems unwilling to accommodate your wishes, especially if no alternative doctor is available. You can usually avoid this kind of confrontation if you communicate well during your pregnancy and are willing to negotiate.

The medical records and nursing notes that are kept in your file during pregnancy and your hospital stay, contain information that is rightfully yours. The paper on which it is recorded belongs to the doctor or hospital, but you have a right to know what the record says about your condition. Many pregnant women are given a copy of their pregnancy record chart to carry with them at all times, in case some unforeseen emergency occurs and treatment is needed away from home. You should ask for an explanation of anything written in your record that you don't understand.

After the birth, you may like to request a copy of your medical record so that you can refer to it later if the need arises. You may move or change doctors before you have your next baby, so a copy of your medical record could be useful to your new caregiver. You should be able to refer to your medical and nursing notes while you are in the hospital as they are usually hung on the end of your bed or kept in the nurses' station in the ward. Once you leave hospital you will need to approach the Administration department and make arrangements to photocopy the material you want. There will probably be a charge for this service.

If complications arise during the labour or birth or the baby is sick and in need of special care, you will have many questions and will want to accumulate as much information as you can about the situation, for future reference. This can be hard to do when you are not feeling well or are in a state of shock following unexpected events. If you don't feel able to pursue the information, your general practitioner can gain access to your medical file and request the information for you.

When you are in labour you will be attended by the midwife and doctor and perhaps one or two assistants. If you are giving birth in a teaching hospital, then you may also be seen by student midwives or doctors. As part of their training, they must attend a number of births to add to their experience, and this is why some mothers find a number of strangers present as the baby is being born. Many women find this sudden influx of students rather alarming, and as a patient you always have the right to ask them to leave, even if you are a hospital patient. If you are a private patient you should always be asked if you mind the extra audience before they are allowed in.

You also have the same rights as a patient in the ante-natal or post-natal wards of the hospital. In teaching hospitals, you may be seen by a number of doctors, usually residents or registrars, who are doing specialised training. They should ask permission to attend you, particularly if you are a private patient, and they should introduce themselves so you know who they are. Ask for their names if necessary. You have the right to ask for another opinion or referral to the supervising obstetrician if necessary.

If you are a hospital patient, and receive your ante-natal care through the outpatient clinic, you still have rights as a patient. Your main problem will be that it is unlikely that you will see the same midwives and doctors at each clinic visit unless the clinic is arranged on a team basis with the same group of caregivers seeing the same clients each time. With clinic care and the changing roster of staff it is very useful to make a note of the name of the doctor or midwife you see at each visit and the advice you were given. With the lack of continuity of care, you can be given conflicting advice and confused messages about your condition. If a problem develops, then try to see the same person each time so that they can build up a clear picture of your case. Each ante-natal clinic is presided over by a specialist obstetrician and you can always ask to see this person if you are dissatisfied with your care in the clinic. If you want to obtain a second opinion, it can sometimes be done by attending the clinic on a different day, when another team is in attendance.

When you are pregnant, you are responsible for the health and well-being not only of yourself but also of your baby. Your doctor or midwife has a professional responsibility to take appropriate care of you, but it is up to you to make the final decisions on matters that affect you or the baby directly. This may seem difficult at times, but as soon as the baby is born you will be fully responsible anyway. You are just exercising your rights and responsibilities a little earlier!

Medical matters often seem mysterious and complicated, but it should be possible to obtain a clear explanation so you can be fully involved at all times. Indeed, it is your right to know what is happening to you and to have the labour and birth managed in the way you desire. You can seek advice from many sources, but ultimately it will be up to you to make the decisions, and even though this may be hard, it will help you to fully appreciate and accept the final outcome.

PART 2

9

Making labour easier

This section is directed primarily to the support people who will be with the mother during her labour. In making support people the focus of this section, it is hoped that the labouring woman will be assured of the help she needs to labour effectively and that you will feel confident and secure in your role. Of course, the information will be of interest to the mother too, and it may help to explain some of the feelings and needs that may be experienced in labour.

So, for all of you who plan to be with a woman during her labour, these suggestions are for you!

A labouring woman has instincts to guide her though the birth process and if she can tune in to her body she will discover what she needs to do to speed the birth and ease the pain. She will gradually withdraw into herself as labour proceeds and communicate less and less so that she can focus all her attention on her body's actions and the baby within.

As support people, your primary task is to provide her with an environment in which these instincts can be acknowledged and expressed. You will need to be sensitive to the changes in her behaviour and resourceful in providing care and assistance. This is easier than it seems and you can make a very positive contribution to her experience of birth.

A woman in labour has some very basic needs.

Privacy Labour works best when the mother can tap into the instinctive birthing behaviour that is imprinted in her brain. She will find it easier to tap into her instincts if she feels unobserved: she should not be inhibited by the presence of onlookers, so privacy is of basic importance.

Time Labour should flow in a rhythmical way with an increasing tempo as time goes on. It is a very individual process and women vary in the time they need to give birth. The first birth usually takes longer than other labours as the body has to learn its role and perform the task for the first time. No woman should be hurried or reminded in any way of the time during labour. Since labours vary so much, there are no firm guidelines, only many examples.

Protection A woman in labour is very vulnerable to outside influences that could slow down her labour. This is part of the survival mechanism provided by nature to ensure that the new baby doesn't arrive into a dangerous place. She needs to feel protected and secure from any threat to her safety or privacy.

Permission A woman in labour must feel that she can be herself in a completely free way. She needs to feel that those helping her are not embarrassed or frightened by her behaviour, but have a deep understanding that women may need to behave in a variety of ways to ease the pain and speed the process.

Peace of mind A labouring mother needs to know that she is ready to labour; that she will not be disturbed as she gives birth; that those who are with her understand and respect her needs; what will happen as the labour proceeds and that she can give birth as nature intends. Good preparation will lay the foundations for this peace of mind and her support people will help provide the rest as the birth proceeds.

Your role as a support person will have been established during the pregnancy. Together with the mother you will have planned for the arrival of the baby and readied yourself for the tasks ahead. With all the preliminary organisation completed, you are now awaiting that exciting moment when you realise that the labour has begun, and the baby is on its way into your arms. Now a new phase in your relationship with her is unfolding, and you can look forward to an exhilarating and emotional time over the next few hours.

Her behaviour during labour: what you will see

The way a woman behaves in labour will be very individual, yet she will give you signals that will help tell you which stage of labour she is in. You can use these signposts to assess progress and to determine what will help her at this time. As you accompany your partner through labour you will begin to understand her particular way of giving birth and this will help you to develop sensitivity to those nuances in her behaviour that tell you something new is happening or that a change is occurring. Practical suggestions as to what you can do for the mother at various stages of labour are given in Chapter 11.

As labour begins

It is sometimes difficult to tell when a mother begins to labour. Strong Braxton–Hicks contractions which come frequently and sometimes painfully may be interpreted as the start of labour. These are really only 'practice' contractions and genuine labour does have a different feel. Therefore, it may be wise to wait until some of the other signs appear before deciding that labour really is underway.

There will be various signs that labour is starting.

- Contractions begin, usually mild at first and often irregularly spaced. As each contraction begins it will increase in intensity to a peak before subsiding. This wave-like feeling is the main difference from the Braxton–Hicks contractions of pregnancy, which have a consistent intensity without any peaks. Some mothers, however, go straight into heavy labour with little warning, and find that contractions come strongly and quickly. This is more likely to happen if this is a second or subsequent baby.

- Backache, which is usually intermittent, is commonly caused by the contractions being registered in her back rather than at the front of her tummy.

- Membranes break, releasing the amniotic fluid from in front of the baby's head. This happens at the beginning of about 15% of labours, and more often if the baby is in a posterior position in the mother's pelvis (that is, the baby is facing forwards, not towards the mother's back as it usually does). If the membranes break completely, there will be a gush of fluid of about half to one cup in all. If the membranes break only partially, a leak will occur and the slow dribble may be confused with urine. You can smell the difference if you collect the fluid on a pad. Leaking in this way is not a very reliable sign that labour is starting, and you should wait to see what other signs develop. Contact your midwife or doctor if in doubt.

- A mucous plug may appear from the vagina, or a heavy mucous 'show', tinged with blood. This is easy to miss and is not a reliable sign of labour starting. It means that the cervix is beginning to soften and that labour will probably begin in the next few hours, days or perhaps next week!

- Diarrhoea may be noticed as the bowels empty to make more room for the descending baby.

- Vague feelings arise that something is happening: perhaps twinges, heightened emotions, energetic 'nesting' behaviour or other mild internal signals that labour is about to begin. Experienced mothers will probably be more aware of these signs than the first-time mother.

At the start of labour, when the contractions are mild and well spaced, you will notice very little change in her normal appearance and behaviour. Emotional reactions may include excitement, apprehension, relief that the waiting is over, anticipation and even panic! As time passes, however, these initial reactions tend to settle and a pattern for coping with the labour will begin to emerge. She will probably be able to continue with her normal daily activities for some time in these early stages, provided that she takes care not to tire herself. Sometimes, if the early part of labour is prolonged, a feeling of boredom can develop together with an impatience for something to happen. Some women get anxious if they think progress is too slow at this time, but anxiety will itself cause the labour to slow down, especially in the early phase. Encouragement and distraction can be useful to counteract these feelings and help the labour to establish strongly. Progress will come soon enough!

As first stage develops

As labour goes on there will be gradual signs that the cervix is beginning to dilate and the baby is moving further down into the pelvis.

- The contractions will become more regular and closer together. Remember that it is the length and strength of each contraction that indicates progress, not the space between them. Although contractions usually get closer together, some women find their contractions always come at regular intervals, with a gradual strengthening of each contraction and an increase in their intensity and painfulness over time.
- A pattern and rhythm may develop, incorporating the rise and fall of the contractions, the complete break between and the settling of the mother into a routine that allows her comfort and security.
- She will begin to withdraw into herself, becoming less aware of her surroundings and less willing to talk or respond to others. She may become rather passive, fixed in a comfortable position and unwilling to move. She may indicate her needs by grunting or pointing rather than by using words and she will appreciate having her needs anticipated.
- Some women prefer to remain active, walking or pacing through the contractions. The pelvic rocking and movement can help the baby to descend and the upright posture makes the labour less painful. Try to encourage her to rest between contractions to conserve her energy.

- As first stage continues, she may begin to feel tired, complain of aching legs and want to sit or kneel. Many women get down on the floor at this time, leaning over pillows or furniture for support.
- Most mothers automatically close their eyes as labour advances, to avoid distractions and help them to concentrate on the sensations within their bodies. As she withdraws and focuses inwards, avoid asking questions or making eye contact that will hamper her inner trip towards birth.
- Nausea, shaking, vomiting, passing wind and burping are all common side effects of the developing labour. Thirst and the need to empty the bladder and perhaps bowels also need to be recognised. She will need privacy at these times.

Transition

After some time in first stage, during which you will have become accustomed to her pattern of behaviour, you will begin to see some signs of a change: indications that the labour is entering another phase, called transition. At this time, her uterus starts to alter its action, from opening the cervix (which in most cases is now almost fully open) to the pushing action needed to help expel the baby.

The transitional phase can be brief, just one or two contractions, or prolonged, especially if the dilatation of the cervix has been uneven, and a lip of cervix remains in front of the baby's head.

You will know when this stage has been reached as all women tend to respond to these changes, even if very fleetingly. You may notice any or all of the following occurring.

- The contractions are becoming much longer, stronger and closer together. They are painful, overwhelming and difficult to cope with. Some have two peaks instead of one, and some contractions never seem to fade at all, giving the impression of one long painful contraction lasting some minutes.
- The mother becomes noisy, grunting, shouting, even screaming to relieve some of the tension she is feeling. She needs privacy and to feel uninhibited at this time, which will pass more quickly if she is free to shout out.
- Feelings of fear, desperation and hopelessness being expressed. Negative thoughts ('I want to die', 'Just get the baby out', 'Give me a caesarian') are very common and seem to be a normal reaction to the confrontation with the life force that many women unconsciously experience. There is no need to reassure her, or to convince her she is well and safe: having spoken her

fears she will be quickly able to move into the positive phase of second stage, and will forget these words and feelings afterwards.

- Irrational comments, sudden mood swings, verbal abuse, crying and demands for pain relief (even though it is too late for drugs) are also commonly heard at this time. They are less obvious examples of the natural fear felt by most women during transition, that needs expression rather than suppression.
- A feeling of restlessness, of needing to move or wriggle in response to the huge, powerful contractions at this time. Some mothers find it hard to get comfortable in any position, others find they become immobile, even though they are desperately uncomfortable.
- She may become hot and want to throw off any clothes that are restricting or inhibiting her movements.
- The nausea, shaking and vomiting can become intense or may appear for the first time. She may need to empty her bowels or urinate in response to the increasing pelvic pressure caused by the baby's head.
- At the peak of contractions she may involuntarily catch her breath as preliminary signs of the pushing urge. She may just sound different, making more grunts and straining sounds during contractions. These changes in her noises are a good sign that second stage is beginning.

After some time, which could last from a few minutes to an hour or more, the transitional stage will pass and with it will go the turbulence and negativity she has been feeling. She will appear calmer, less irrational and more like she has been during the earlier phases of labour. It will be a relief to you all!

Second stage

This is the best part of labour, as you will be aware that the baby is about to arrive and all the hard work and waiting during the labour is about to end. With the arrival of second stage you will notice the following.

- She will have involuntary urges to push, lasting 5 or 6 seconds during the contractions.
- The contractions will become shorter (about a minute long) and more spaced apart. Sometimes they may stop altogether at the beginning of second stage, perhaps for some time. If she has such a break, then it is an ideal time to rest, have a drink and

gather strength for the active part of second stage which will come soon.

- She may suddenly feel the urge to empty her bowels, as the baby's head presses deeply into her pelvis. She will need privacy and a suitable place in which to succumb to these sensations—the toilet or a bedpan will help. It is normal to pass some faeces during the birth.
- Sudden surges of activity can occur, as can the need to be upright and to grasp somebody or something. She may drop to the floor, spreading her legs with each push, grasping for support as the baby squeezes down the birth canal. If she is unable to get upright and take her weight on her legs (the preferred position for birth) then she may curl her toes up and pull her knees apart as though she was standing.
- She may need to move around between contractions—to stand up if squatting, sit back if kneeling or walk around to help the baby's descent. You may see involuntary pelvic rocking as she works to ease the baby out.
- Her sounds will change: deep grunts, moans and even high pitched 'singing' may be heard. Screaming usually indicates pain from an outside source—someone touching her vagina, excessive pressure on the perineum because of her birth position, pressure on her sacrum or coccyx if she is sitting or lying. Normal birthing sounds are almost sexual in nature and have no edge of alarm in their tone.
- She will probably have her eyes tightly closed as she marshals all her efforts to push the baby out. If she opens her eyes she will be distracted from her task, so avoid eye contact or questions that require a response.
- Beads of perspiration will form on her flushed face. Giving birth is hot work due to the hormones and the effort involved.
- As the baby is about to crown, some mothers like to touch the head in the vagina, to make contact and give a sense of purpose to the painful stretching sensations of the perineum.

These are the signs that will tell you and the midwife that second stage is underway. They often give a better indication of progress than an assessment made by manually checking the dilatation of the cervix. Some mothers dilate very rapidly towards the end, especially if this is a second or subsequent baby, so behavioural signs give a more reliable indication of the stage of labour than using vaginal examinations alone. Internal checks are also disturbing and uncomfortable, so unless she specifically requests one, they should be avoided.

After the birth

Once the baby is born, the events of the labour will fade a little as all attention is centred on the new baby. Elation, joy, fatigue, relief, excitement, wonder and amazement are typical of the reactions you may experience. It is a special time, vital in the establishment of close ties and successful breastfeeding. Until the placenta is born, the birth will not quite be over and nor is your role finished. You should still be aware of the mother's needs.

- The mother's attention is entirely focused on her baby. She may be uninterested in your reaction or that of the others around her. She has eyes only for this tiny being that she has created, and she needs to take her time to drink in the baby's being, personality and reactions.

- She may not want to hold her baby immediately. Mothers sometimes like to be able to see the baby as a whole for a few moments before lifting it to the breast. It is easiest to do this when sitting upright with the baby lying on its side between her legs. You don't have to pick the baby up immediately—she will gather it to her when she is ready.

- There will be some bleeding with the arrival of the baby, a gush of amniotic fluid and some further mild contractions as the placenta separates and is delivered. You may need to hold the baby for a few moments while the mother sits, kneels or squats to deliver the placenta. There will be a little more bleeding, which should stop once the placenta arrives.

- She may have a 'high' that lasts for hours or days after the birth. The labour hormones will give her energy and a feeling of euphoria.

  If the labour has been long and difficult or was unexpectedly short however, she may feel tired and emotional and be unwilling to see or hold the baby for a while. This will pass in time, and she should still have close access to the baby, who will help her to bond, and to come to terms with the experience.

- Soon after the birth the baby will make some sucking actions and will be ready to nurse at the breast. The mother will need help to sit up to feed the baby and to get properly positioned. As she nurses the baby, some strong contractions may be felt as the uterus contracts in response to the hormones released while nursing. A gush of blood will accompany these contractions, which will diminish in intensity over the first few days.

- The new baby will be alert and awake for some time after the birth. The pupils will be dilated, and they can see you and hear

your voice. A darkened room and quiet privacy will help you all
to get acquainted.

- The mother will probably not want to be separated from her
  baby in the first few days. Weighing the baby, bathing, and routine checks can be safely delayed for at least an hour after the
  birth if the baby is well. Having constant contact will make
  breastfeeding easier to establish, and the mother will rest better
  knowing that the baby is close by her side.
- There is a need to talk over the events of the labour and birth
  with all those who were present. The labour hormones tend to
  dull a woman's memory of these events, and she often likes to fill
  in the gaps by talking to others, especially you and the midwife.
- A few days after the birth, you may notice that she is weepy and
  a little depressed. This is known as the 'three day blues' and is a
  normal reaction to the withdrawal of the endorphins that have
  been in her body over the past nine months. It will pass in 24 to
  48 hours. Give her privacy and let her know she has permission
  to cry or express her emotions.

These are some examples of the range of reactions that women have
during labour. Keep in mind that it is impossible to predict how
long labour will take or how any mother will respond to the rigours
and stresses of labour.

10

Variations

There are as many variations in births as there are women having babies. However, some of the variations are relatively common and could be described as fitting a more general pattern. There are suggestions on ways of helping a mother having one of these labours in the next chapter.

Slow labours

Some women find that labour is slow and tedious, with little progress and much frustration. Sometimes the contractions can be weak and ineffective and other times dilatation is slow despite strong and painful contractions.

If the contractions are weak or intermittent, birth can take several days. Usually the mother is taking her time to enter into established labour and until this happens, the contractions come and go either in an irregular pattern or as gentle regular tightenings that cause little discomfort. Impatience and frustration are common problems, but there is no need to become anxious that something is wrong. Mothers having these types of labours can often carry on with daily activities and will find that eventually they develop strong regular contractions and, after a few hours of concerted effort, give birth well. It is as if her body is taking its time to adjust to labour, and it doesn't need to be rushed. One advantage of this pattern is that there is plenty of warning that the baby is on its way, and there is little chance that the birth will happen unexpectedly!

Sometimes the labour can be long and drawn out, even with painful, hard contractions. The cervix dilates slowly or even stops dilating for a time, while the mother works hard to weather the pain and frustration and inevitable fatigue. This kind of labour may be caused by an unusual position of the baby, such as being breech or posterior, or having its head extended rather than tucked neatly into the pelvis. Anxiety is a major problem for the mother and her support people, as the labour appears to be going nowhere. The attitude of the staff can be crucial in helping the mother to progress, whilst reassurance and careful explanation of what is happening can help reduce anxiety. If the mother starts to panic or become fearful during the first part of labour then the whole process will be slowed and her pain will increase. This in turn will tend to make her more anxious and the cervix can stop dilating altogether.

Very fast labours

Some women find that their labour is very fast, to the point of being tumultuous and overwhelming. Instead of a steady increase in the intensity and strength of contractions over a number of hours, labour begins with the sudden onset of long painful contractions, closely spaced and often accompanied by the sudden breaking of the waters. It feels like being thrown into the deep end of a swimming pool when you can't swim—a combination of panic, struggling to stay on top of the sensations and a strong desire to seek a safe place for the baby's arrival. Short labours are rarely comfortable or enjoyable and some mothers find that afterwards it takes some hours or days before they can understand and accept what happened. Some find that they are in such a state of shock, they don't want to hold or see the baby for a while after the birth.

A labour that is progressing very fast rarely presents any physical problems for either the baby or the mother. It is as if the mother's body just opens up and allows the baby to fall out—often little pushing is needed and tearing of the vagina is uncommon. The baby is usually healthy and unsurprised by its rapid arrival and is often ready to suck right away. Sometimes the placenta delivers quickly too, but it may take some time to detach before it arrives to complete the birth process.

A very fast labour may mean that the baby arrives before you make it to the hospital. Although you will feel panicky and anxious remember that a fast easy labour like this rarely presents a problem for mother or baby. You need to do very little.

- Try to find a safe, quiet place—in the bathroom or toilet if you are at home, off to the side of the road away from traffic and onlookers if you are on the way to the hospital.
- Keep the baby warm by wrapping it up and give it to the mother to hold.
- Keep the mother sitting up to help the placenta to separate.
- Don't cut the cord—leave it undisturbed. If the placenta comes

out, wrap it separately but keep it next to the baby.
* Make your way to the hospital when you are ready, or phone and ask someone to visit you at home.

Backache labours

Constant back pain usually indicates that the baby is in a posterior position and is pressing on the mother's sacrum making her back ache during labour. The baby will need to turn through almost 180 degrees to be born and this will take time. Any long labour characterised by backache will probably indicate that the baby is in this position, but the midwife can confirm your suspicions if you are unsure.

When you are helping a mother with this kind of labour you will find that fatigue is a major problem. The labour hormones, especially endorphins, will help the mother to manage the pain, but as time goes by and she begins to tire, it will be less easy for her to cope. The rate of dilatation of the cervix is often slow due to the less favourable position of the baby's head and this adds to the problem of fatigue.

Complications

Nature has designed the birth process to work smoothly and efficiently, to give the baby the best possible start in life and the mother a rewarding and satisfying experience. Labour should be straightforward for most women: approximately 90 per cent should give birth well if they have the right surroundings and support.

Occasionally something does go wrong; perhaps the labour slows or stops and affects the baby; the baby finds the process distressing; there may be mechanical problems such as the baby being too big to fit through the pelvis easily. The chances of these situations developing are reduced if there are no attempts made to modify or change the labour from its natural pattern. Induction, rupturing the membranes artificially, administering pain killing drugs and using electronic fetal monitoring are all ways of disturbing labour that can lead to the development of complications. If you can help reduce the mother's reliance on these obstetric interventions she will have a better chance of producing a healthy baby after a fulfilling labour.

If a problem does develop before or during labour, a mother will often be aware herself that something is wrong, even if this is her first experience of birth. Women can sometimes sense that the baby is stuck or in trouble, and their feelings on these matters should be respected and investigated. In this situation, any mother will happily accept, even demand, some form of help, and she should have your total support.

Your role at this time will be to help and protect her, while making every effort to relieve the situation with a minimum of physical and emotional trauma. Some suggestions on how to do this are in the next chapter. If a complication does develop, her behaviour will change, and you could see the following.

- Confusion, concern and worry about what is happening. Instead of being engrossed in the labour, with eyes closed and reduced external contact with others, she may be anxious, agitated and focused on her helpers, particularly the doctor, at this time.
- Impatience. The desire to get help quickly becomes paramount. Her attitude to the labour changes, and it is seen as an impediment to the safe arrival of the baby.
- The labour hormones are still having an effect on her behaviour. She may have difficulty thinking clearly or making decisions. In a crisis with the baby, most women immediately relinquish all responsibility for making decisions to the doctor, and while his professional guidance is vitally important, she still needs to have a role in making the decisions. This will help her accept the unexpected outcome of the labour more easily when it is all over.
- She will probably be asked to remain on the bed as she is readied for the necessary medical procedures. If she has been mobile and upright until now, lying down will be painful and uncomfortable in contrast. The sudden increase in pain may frighten and confuse her further.
- Her attitude to her labour often changes. Instead of seeing her body's labours as a positive effort directed towards giving her the long-awaited baby, she may feel negative, seeing her body as an enemy wilfully inflicting pain on her. The baby and its needs can be pushed aside in this change of heart and, having abandoned her natural coping mechanisms, she focuses on her own misery and desire to obtain relief at any cost. This change of attitude can be confusing for support people to grasp, and you should be aware of any conflict in your own feelings at this time, so you can be positive in your support for her decisions.

Whenever a complication develops in the pregnancy or labour, it is natural for all concerned to become anxious and fearful for the baby, and the mother. The inevitable change in plans, the necessary deviation from the pre-arranged birth plan, the shift in expectations can all create confusion, anger, insecurity and dependence on others rather than yourselves. The over-riding concern is to produce a healthy baby and personal needs and desires are often subordinated to this desired outcome. You will see and feel a range of emotions and reactions in these circumstances, all of which are valid. The more you can accept and understand them, the better will be the overall experience even if your plans turn out unexpectedly.

11

Practical suggestions for labour support people

Once labour begins, your task as a support person will truly begin. Your aim is to help your partner labour easily, effectively and with a minimum of pain. Although she has the resources within herself that she needs to labour well, your job is to make it as easy as possible for her to tap into these hidden talents. If she labours and gives birth using her own instincts, the natural hormones she will produce will protect her from excessive pain and ensure the health of the baby. To have a healthy baby and a happy mother is everyone's aim at this time.

Your position at the mother's side during labour is very special and of great importance. Through your efforts she will find the time and space that she needs and will feel confident in allowing her body to work in its own way to give birth. Your calm and quiet presence will enhance her experience and help allay her fears and anxieties. Birth may be an unknown quantity, like taking a journey through uncharted territory, but it has the power and potential to reveal exciting insights and provide untold rewards for you both.

If this is the first time you have been asked to assist a woman in labour, you will probably feel unsure of your role and at a loss to know what practical help you can offer. The suggestions outlined below are intended as a guide. You will find further information in *Preparing for Birth*, especially on the nature of labour, the drugs and medical interventions available and the positions she might find comfortable. The following ideas are intended to help you develop a concept of labour support as well as offering practical pointers.

Homebirth

If you are planning a homebirth, many of the following suggestions will be useful for you to try. Obviously, the comments related to managing in hospital will not apply, unless you are transferred for some reason. In this case there will probably be a problem, and the section on handling complications may be most relevant.

Even though you are in an ideal environment for birth, you should still be aware of the mother's need for privacy, time, and as few disturbances as possible. A common problem with birth at home is having too many people present. This may also extend to your other children, and it is hard to predict the effects of having a crowd, even if they are all apparently involved and integral to the experience. The need to be alone, to confront the strength and power of birth by herself, is often of prime importance to a woman at this time, and giving her this kind of space and time, especially in the beneficial atmosphere of home, will make the birth quicker, easier, and therefore safer.

When labour starts

Make sure that she has someone nearby at all times. If you are at work when she begins labour, alert a neighbour or friend to stay with her if it will take you some time to get home. A labouring woman doesn't need to have someone watching her constantly, but she needs to know that there is someone within easy reach in case of sudden need.

Phone your extra support people so they can arrange to be with you when you need them. If it is early evening or during the night, they can get some extra sleep in readiness for their involvement. A well-rested, fresh support person will be able to relieve you later on when you need a break.

Put her bag for the hospital and the labour aids you plan to take to the hospital in the car right away. Check on the whereabouts of your pets, lock the doors and windows, and then you will be ready to leave the house whenever she wants to go, without a last minute rush. Check you have packed her pregnancy record card, health insurance details, Medicare number, and have small change for phone calls.

If you are staying at home for the birth, phone the midwife and tell her that labour has begun. She will tell you when to expect her and answer any questions you may have.

Have something light and easy to eat. It may have been many hours since your last full meal and it may be some time before you get the next one, so make a simple meal to keep everyone's energy level up. A nourishing drink, soup, toast, eggs, or a sandwich would be suitable, but be guided by her requests. As labour progresses she will feel less like eating, but keep offering her drinks at regular intervals.

Suggest a shower: to freshen up, wash hair and generally feel relaxed and awake. You too might benefit from a hot shower at this time! A long shower or bath, however, will probably slow the labour down in the early phases, so keep it brief.

Get her comfortable in an upright position that will help the baby descend and lessen the pain. It may be hours before the labour establishes strongly and in the meantime, she needs to conserve energy and rest. If she can sleep, then this will help, but most women in labour find sleeping impossible. Prop her up with pillows and offer the television or music to while away the time. Gentle exercise such as ironing is favoured by some women and forms part of the 'nesting' behaviour. Long walks and tiring activity should be avoided: you will both need energy later and it is not helpful to enter the accelerated phase of labour already exhausted.

Many women labour most effectively on their own, with help nearby. Even at this early stage, some women may like to spend some time alone, perhaps on the toilet (useful if diarrhoea is present!) or walking in the garden. This allows a mental space to think of the baby and get ready for the transition to motherhood.

There is no need to watch a labouring woman closely to make sure that she is alright. Having people staring or watching intently can be very disturbing and inhibiting. Casual observation, together with a listening ear for the sounds she makes will tell you how she is feeling. Stand beside or behind her not facing her as this will lessen her impression that she is being watched.

If labour begins at night, keep the lights low to encourage restfulness. You will both be missing out on sleep and so any reminder that this is normally a time for rest will help you to conserve energy. If it is daytime when she goes into labour, draw the curtains to help her feel cosy and safe in the darkened room.

If the membranes have ruptured, there will be a trickle of amniotic fluid every time she has a contraction. She will feel safer and more secure with some pads and panties to catch the drips. Women generally feel less vulnerable if they can remain covered during the early part of labour, and perhaps all the way through. She may feel embarrassed at having others change pads for her, so give her privacy so she can do this for herself (for example, in the toilet).

Keep her warm during labour. Feet often get cold so woolly socks will be welcome. A dressing gown or large T-shirt that covers her fully will help her to feel secure and warm, especially in the early first stage.

Try and reduce any distractions in her immediate environment. If there is unavoidable noise nearby, try giving her some favourite music through headphones to block the unwelcome sounds. Taking a shower will reduce the impact of outside noise. Take the phone off the hook too.

Going to hospital

The ideal time to take her to hospital is when she says she wants to go. While most first time mothers will be happiest and labour best at home for some time in first stage, she may feel uncomfortable about staying too long and prefer to go to the place where she will give birth right at the beginning. Be guided by her, and try not to push her into going when you want to take her!

The responsibility of supporting a labouring woman can weigh heavily, particularly for a man who can never be familiar with the sensations and emotions that characterise labour. It is often the father who wants the mother to go to hospital so he can be reassured that all is well and be supported by the midwife. If you have been able to arrange for another support person, especially another woman to be with you in labour, then being able to share the emotional load with another will often make staying at home more comfortable for you.

If this is not the first baby, the labour will be shorter than the first time, and the mother may indicate quite quickly once she is labour that now is the time to go to the hospital. Don't be lulled into a false sense of security because the first labour was long and there was plenty of time. The mother will know even better this time when she wants to make her move from home, so you will need to be ready to move quickly (but calmly!).

The trip to the hospital is always uncomfortable for a woman in labour. You can make it a little easier for her if you make her comfortable in the back of the car, leaning forward over some pillows or the back seat, if there is space. Have some clean, old towels in the car to mop up the fluid should the membranes break, and a plastic container with a lid, in case she feels sick. Positioning her forward over pillows or on hands and knees will help slow the labour down, and this will help her to feel more secure. Cover her with a blanket or towel so she feels less exposed, attach the seat belt as best you can and drive carefully to the hospital.

When you arrive at the hospital, your first stop will be the admissions desk. You should know where to find this from your explorations during the pregnancy or on the hospital tour. It is unlikely that you can leave your car at the main entrance for any length of time, so once you have her safely inside and the paperwork complete, move your car quickly so you can accompany her to the labour ward.

Stay with her at all times. It is unlikely that you will be asked to leave while admission procedures are being carried out, but some hospital staff still like to ask the fathers and extra support people to wait outside. This is unreasonable and she needs your support at all times, particularly when settling into the unfamiliar setting of the hospital. If she requests that you stay, then her wishes should be accepted by the staff.

There are a variety of admission procedures that need to be done, including weighing, testing urine, an internal examination, measuring blood pressure, taking her temperature, listening to the baby's heart beat and feeling the baby's position in her tummy. Shaves and enemas are rarely offered these days as they have been proven unnecessary. All these procedures should have been covered in your pre-natal class and should be explained by the midwife at the time. Routine electronic fetal heart rate monitoring, insertion of an intra-venous drip and rupturing of membranes are all optional and should be carefully considered before you accept them. They are not necessary unless there is already an obvious medical problem with the baby.

Once the admission procedures have been completed, she will be shown to the room where she will labour and give birth. Sometimes there is a 'first stage room' or lounge area with comfortable chairs and perhaps a television. You should be aware of your hospital's arrangements from the information you were given on your hospital tour.

Make the mother and yourself feel at home. Unpack your labour aids and rearrange the furniture in the room to make it as comfortable as possible. Push the bed to the side to make more room if it seems cramped, and locate the light switches so you can dim the lights. Check in the drawers and cupboards to find the spare pads and a vomit bowl, in case of need. There should be water and a glass, but if not, ask for it to be provided.

The labour ward should have bean bags and floor mats available as well as extra pillows. If you can't find them in the room, ask the midwife to bring some for you. As labour progresses, many mothers want to kneel down on the floor, leaning over pillows or a bean bag. Put a sheet over the bean bag to make it more comfortable and use a sheet on the mat too, to catch drips and eliminate the vinyl feel under foot.

Find out where the toilet and shower are. Many hospitals have limited facilities and they are often located at an inconvenient distance from most of the labour wards. If you are in a birth centre, a bathroom will be nearby. If the toilet is too far away to be convenient, then the mother will need to use a bedpan frequently.

Find out where these are kept so that you don't need to wait for a midwife to get one, if the need is urgent. Find out where the kitchen or tea making facilities are so that you can get yourself some refreshments when you need them. In some hospitals, morning and afternoon tea are available in labour wards as part of the regular meal service. Most hospitals have a kiosk where light refreshments can be bought, but this won't be open during the night! It is best to take your own food and drink so you can be sure you can get a drink or snack at any time: some sandwiches and a thermos of hot tea or coffee will be useful.

There will be a number of staff on duty who should introduce themselves to you and explain their role. Most will be wearing a name tag, but if not make sure you ask their name. Introduce yourself and the rest of the support team and explain what assistance you would like during the labour. There will be staff changes in the early morning (about 7.00 a.m.), again in the late afternoon (around 3.00 p.m.) and at night (about 11.00 p.m.) There is a period at each of these times where the staff on each shift overlap so that smooth handing over can take place. If your baby will be born very close to the arrival of the new shift and you have become attached to the midwife who is about to go off duty, you could request that she stay to help at the birth. This is sometimes possible and it is good to have familiar people with you at the climax of the labour.

The midwife will phone the doctor when you arrive at the hospital to give him the first progress report. The midwife will continue to pass on information about progress throughout the labour. The doctor will aim to arrive when second stage has begun (or a little before if this is your second or subsequent baby). It is unlikely that the doctor will see you during the labour as a matter of course. If she is present in the hospital at the time, perhaps to see other patients, then a visit may be made to assess the mother personally. (If the labour is being induced, however, the doctor should be there to begin the labour, set up the drip, rupture the membranes and check that the labour is underway.) If there is a problem at any time during the labour, the doctor will be summoned immediately to assist. If he is not immediately available, then another doctor or the registrar may be called to help if it is an emergency.

During first stage

From time to time, the midwife will perform a number of routine observations to check on progress and the baby's well-being. These checks include listening to the baby's heartbeat through a trumpet-shaped stethoscope or an amplified ultrasound stethoscope, taking the mother's blood pressure and temperature, and timing the contractions to gauge their strength. Every few hours, an internal examination to assess the amount of dilatation of the cervix may be suggested. The most important test is the noting of the baby's heartbeat, as this gives a good indication of how the baby is faring through the labour. An experienced midwife knows, just through observation, how much progress a mother is making during labour and this can reduce her need to disturb the mother to make more formal examinations, especially internal assessments.

As labour settles into a pattern, your main task will be to help provide the mother with her basic needs in labour: privacy, time, emotional support, practical soothing help, peace of mind and permission to do whatever she likes. She will be unaware of the hours passing and a routine will probably develop with you quietly attending to her needs as she labours on. This may be the pattern for many hours, until a change in her behaviour indicates that the transition phase between first and second stage has been reached.

Keep disturbing influences away. Ask extra staff to leave or hold conversations outside rather than allowing discussion to carry on around her during labour. The midwife will have to check progress regularly, but this can be done quietly without disturbing the mother's position. Avoid small talk: this is no time to discuss the tennis or football!

Comfort aids you can offer during first stage

Make the room as dark, quiet and cosy as you can. Put a mat on the floor and heap up pillows or a bean bag so that she can get comfortable. A chair may be useful, especially one without arms, so she can sit on it back to front and lean over its back with her head on a pillow. Encourage her to make herself comfortable away from the door, so that when it is opened she is not visible to others passing outside.

Check the way she looks once she has settled.

- Is her head supported? Use extra pillows to allow her to rest.
- Are her feet fully resting on the floor or does she have her heels up? Put a rolled pillow under each foot or use two footstools or something similar to take the pressure from under her thighs.
- Are her arms relaxed and floppy? Bent elbows and relaxed shoulders will help her conserve energy and reduce tension.

- Is her face calm? Some gentle massage on her forehead or beside her eyes will help her relax.
- Is her jaw loose and is she breathing slowly in a relaxed manner? Some gentle stroking under her chin will remind her to release any tension in her jaw.
- Is her mouth dry? Sips of water or something to suck (glucose sweets are often good), lip cream and drinks will be welcome.
- Does she have her eyes open? Encourage her to focus her energies within by keeping her eyes closed, especially when labour picks up tempo. If her eyes are open she will be easily distracted and this can slow labour down.
- Is she constantly talking and chattering away? This is fine at the beginning of labour, but as time goes on, she needs to be quiet and self-absorbed. Avoid unnecessary talk and the asking of questions yourself, to allow her to slip into her own world.
- Are her feet warm? Put on some woolly socks.
- Does she look comfortable and confident? Your touch, your reassurance and calm presence will give her strength. Occasional praise and comforting hugs go a long way in labour!

Don't forget other ideas too.

Massage Gentle stroking using your whole hand and relaxed fingers is very soothing. Make each stroke slow and rhythmical and use enough pressure to avoid tickling. Ask her for feedback and adjust your touch accordingly. Using a vegetable oil will help avoid friction and skin damage. Try massaging the back in long strokes, the shoulders and over the arms, the feet, and her face.

Some mothers find that as labour progresses the massaging becomes annoying and they want all direct touch to stop. This can be a surprise to you all, especially if she normally loves being massaged! If this happens try holding her hand or wiping her face from time to time. She will sense your presence and that is often enough.

Holding This is good for relieving tension in specific areas, such as the shoulders, buttocks, or face. Position your hands over the area in question and use a firm pressure for several minutes. The warmth and gentle pressure will help her to release tension in the underlying muscles and it is very calming. Holding her hips on each side can help her to feel that she is still 'together'.

Counter pressure Firm pressure to counter the force of the baby against the pelvis can be very comforting. The need for counter pressure is greatest if the baby is in a posterior position and its head is pressing against the sacrum. Use the heel of both hands, one on top of the other and push against the sore spot, which she will indicate to you, especially during the contractions. The sore spot may move lower down as the baby rotates and descends.

Hot packs Some combination of water and heat is the best form of non-invasive pain relief in labour. There are several types of hot packs you can try, and it is best to take these with you so that you are assured of their availability when you need them.

The hot/cold jelly-filled packs available from the chemist are useful: they can be heated up in very hot water and are flexible enough to mould to any shape required. Hot water bottles are too heavy and inflexible to be of any use in labour.

Another alternative is to use hot, wet cloths (fabric nappies or small hand towels are ideal). You will need a bucket and a pair of rubber gloves to protect your hands. Fill the bucket almost full with very hot water, soak the cloths and as you see a contraction developing, take one out, wring it out firmly, and lay it over the sore area. Leave it there until you replace it with another hot cloth at the beginning of the next contraction. This can provide such a welcome pain relief that it is wise not to start it too soon in labour—leave it until late first stage or you will be wringing out cloths for hours on end!

Baths or showers Not all hospitals have a deep bath, but all will have a shower that can be used to promote relaxation and reduce the pain. Once again, save this very effective pain relieving idea until it is really needed at the end of first stage. Getting in the shower or bath too early can slow the labour down, but if offered at a later stage can help the mother to dilate very quickly. This can also be useful if the rate of dilatation remains static over a number of hours, and could be tried before inserting a drip to speed up the labour.

Leave the mother in the bath or shower for as long as she wants. Have a stool or plastic chair handy so she can lean over it for support in the shower, and a pillow available for her head if she is in the bath. She may still want hot cloths applied in addition to the shower, and may still want your company to hold and support her. Pack a swimsuit for yourself in case of need!

Drinks Labour can be hot and tiring work so she will need regular drinks to relieve her thirst and to give her the energy she needs to labour efficiently. In the early stages, teas, fruit juices or cordials may be welcome. As labour progresses, water will probably be preferred or ice chips if she is feeling nauseous. Some women find flat lemonade is helpful for nausea too. As a rough guide, she needs about one glass of fluid every hour, and may need more in second stage, which can be thirsty work.

'Goody' bag This is a collection of labour aids that you can have ready well in advance to take with you to the hospital. You may not use all these things, but it is better to be well prepared than to find you lack the very item you need to help her during labour. The following list is not meant to be exhaustive, and you can add or subtract any items to suit your own needs.

- comfortable clothes for the labour (large T-shirt for her, tracksuit or similar for you)
- dressing gown, slippers, woolly socks for her; shower hat, swim suit for you
- food and drink
- towels or nappies, bucket and rubber gloves for hot packs
- lip chap, glucose lollies, natural sponge to moisten for her to suck if her mouth is dry
- music, tape recorder and headphones
- camera for the first photos of the baby

Transition

As the transitional time between first and second stage develops you will notice some of the characteristic changes in her behaviour mentioned in Chapter 9. At this time your support will be vital and your confidence and praise will have enormous effect on her well-being. If you are worried about what you are seeing or hearing, ask the midwife for information about what is happening. She can make suggestions and support you, so that you in turn can support the mother. Although the mother may appear out of control and suffering considerable pain, it may be that she is just expressing her feelings and that the turmoil is rapidly passing. Don't throw in the towel yourself! She needs solid support and understanding and if you feel anxious and worried, your emotions will be easily picked up by her, and may add to her own concerns. Leave the room and take a break if you are finding this part of her labour difficult. Make sure that she is being cared for by someone else, perhaps the midwife, while you are away. Anxious, panicking onlookers will slow her labour down and make her passage through this part of labour more difficult than it need be.

What you can do at this time

All of the suggestions in the preceding section are still useful during transition. Since she will probably be restless with much pain and discomfort, a psychological boost from being able to offer something 'new' or different for comfort can make a difference and help overcome any feelings of 'getting nowhere' that she may be having.

At this stage in the labour, pain-killing drugs given to the mother pose risks for the baby and so should not be offered. You will need to be resourceful in finding other ways of reducing her pain. You could try one of the following ideas.

- A hot bath or shower will provide an immediate reduction in pain and give her some activity.
- Hot compresses, such as hot packs or hot wet towels can be applied to painful areas. These are a good standby if a shower or bath is not available.
- Help her into a more comfortable position. Being upright, moving about or pelvic rocking may help to decrease the pressure from the baby on other pelvic structures, encourage descent and aid the last centimetres of dilatation of the cervix.
- A knee-chest position will help more even dilatation if there is an anterior lip of cervix in front of the baby's head.
- She may be shivery and shaky in response to the huge, powerful contractions she is experiencing. Keep her warm, massage shaking limbs firmly and change her position to relieve these symptoms.
- Nausea is often a problem at this time. If she can vomit the nausea will usually settle. Sucking on ice cubes and sipping flat lemonade helps some women.
- Help her to express her feelings—to shout, moan and say what is on her mind. Releasing her emotions and fears will have a positive effect on progress. There is no need for you to constantly reassure her or be frightened by any negative outbursts. If she is abusive, accept that she does not mean it personally, but needs to find a focus for her overwhelming reactions to the strength and power of the labour. The moment will pass, and she will forget most of what happened when the baby is born.
- Allow her the freedom to do as she pleases at this time. Avoid giving her instructions, making suggestions, forcing her to make decisions or interact with anybody until she is ready. This is the most turbulent time of the whole labour and only she can know what it is like. Trust that she will be able to weather the storm

and come through with flying colours. So will you!

Your role in second stage

Once second stage begins, the midwife will be with you constantly, checking the baby's heartbeat, monitoring progress and liaising with the doctor. You will find the midwife a useful ally in ensuring that the mother is allowed to give birth as she wishes. You will also find that the midwife will become the primary support person for the mother, and this will relieve you of some of the responsibility you have had up till now.

There are many useful things you can do at this time.

- Help your partner into an upright, comfortable position. She will know which one allows the most effective pushing but she might need to experiment with several alternative positions to find the right one.
- Try to keep her off the bed during second stage. It will be easier for her to move around, rest between contractions and maintain some autonomy if she is away from the bed and in a place of her choice. Put a mat under her feet or knees on the floor, and be ready to hold her securely during contractions.
- She will still need privacy and to feel that she is not being constantly watched. Having people staring at her genital area can be embarrassing and inhibiting for a mother in labour, and this is less likely to happen if she is not lying on a bed.
- Most women will have their eyes tightly closed during second stage. Don't encourage her to look in a mirror or answer questions at this time. She needs to remain closely in touch with the feeling of the baby in her vagina so she can judge how much to push and when to ease the baby out. Distractions, especially instructions from the midwife or doctor, should be kept to a minimum. If they can't be avoided, try turning her around so that she is facing away from everyone with her eyes closed. The doctor and midwife will still be able to see what is happening, and the risks of disturbance and intervention will be reduced.
- Second stage is a time of activity, in contrast to the more passive first stage. She will move and adjust her body to ease the passage of the baby (provided she is able to be upright and self-supporting) and she will grasp either you or the furniture for support during contractions. It will be tiring holding her weight, so you must rest between contractions too. She will be thirsty, so offer a drink frequently.

When the baby is born

The moment of birth is magical and exciting. The baby arrives, is greeted by everyone and begins to explore its new world. As you meet the baby at last, you may feel that the birth is over, that your role is over and that once the formalities are completed, you can leave the mother and baby for a well earned rest. But there are still some important actions you can take to ensure that the placenta is delivered smoothly, that mother and baby make close contact and that breastfeeding begins well.

When the baby is born, help the mother to sit upright. Don't lie her down which will increase the chances of haemorrhage and slow the arrival of the placenta. If she sits unsupported, she will be in the best position to help the placenta separate and also to see and hold her new baby. If she is tired and insists on lying down, help her to lie on one side, with the baby beside her on the floor mat or the bed.

As soon as the baby shows signs of being interested, encourage the mother to breastfeed. Most mothers will automatically nurse their babies, but if there are many distractions then this may be overlooked and the opportunity and advantages of early breastfeeding may be lost.

Try to give the mother continued privacy for at least the first hour after the birth. When the baby is healthy and strong, there is no need for early cutting of the cord, weighing, bathing, measuring, Vitamin K injections and other newborn procedures to be done right away. These can all wait to be done by the mother's side at a later time. Keep the lights low, the voices quiet and the number of people to a minimum. You can play a vital role in preserving these precious moments as a family.

If she needs stitches, especially following an episiotomy, try to have these done quickly so that she can spend time with baby alone. A small tear may not need a stitch at all and could be safely delayed until a later time.

In the days following the birth, it can be helpful to monitor visitor numbers so that mother and baby are not tired or overly disturbed during the crucial first days together. One way of doing this is to delay announcements of the birth until a few days later, so that only immediate family are involved.

12

Variations in labour

How to help her through a long labour

The first thing for support people to remember is to stay calm and unworried themselves. You will need reassurance and information yourself before you can feel totally comfortable with this kind of drawn-out labour.

- Check with the midwife or doctor to find out what is happening. If she is in early labour, the membranes haven't ruptured and she is still at home, call your childbirth educator or the midwife at the hospital for suggestions and reassurance.
- Some mothers like to visit the hospital to be sure that all is well before they return home to labour in a familiar environment; indeed this is advisable if the membranes have already ruptured. However it is better to be at home rather than in hospital when the early stage of labour is prolonged, as it is easier to have privacy at home and there is less pressure from hospital staff to try and speed up the labour artificially.
- Make sure that she is resting as much as she can and that she is continuing to eat and drink during these early stages. This will help to prevent fatigue which will add to her discomfort later on. Take the phone off the hook, offer her a quiet activity such as the television, radio or music and stay positive!
- If you are at the hospital and the labour is strong with little progress, check for physical reasons for the lack of progress (ask the midwife). If there seems no obvious reason for the lengthy labour such as the baby's head being in a posterior position, then look for sources of anxiety in the mother. Fears, disturbances, lack of privacy or distraction could all be factors in delaying progress. You could try:

  - moving her to a quieter place
  - asking extra people to leave so she has more privacy

- a warm bath or shower
- making her comfortable in the toilet by herself
- darkening the room
- giving her time, thus removing pressure on her to perform to a timetable
- making your comments positive and trying to keep her morale high. Some babies just take their time, so keep optimistic!

To help her through a long backache labour you could try:

- giving her a quiet, dark place
- keeping all noisy distractions, including conversation, to a minimum
- disturbing her as little as possible
- getting her into a comfortable position leaning forward to take the weight of the baby off her back. On the floor is best with a mat under her knees, and offer massage, counter pressure on her lower back, and regular drinks
- helping her into a hot bath or shower from time to time
- hot compresses on her lower back or wherever she needs warmth and support
- helping her to walk around from time to time to aid circulation and the baby's descent

If her labour is slow, sometimes long walks, car rides over bumpy roads, castor oil and other measures that might speed up labour are suggested (ask your midwife). While these may work in some instances, there is always the risk that she will become fatigued, suffer undue discomfort (castor oil is not very pleasant!) and that anxiety will develop if the labour still fails to get moving. Since some mothers always start labour slowly, it may be disadvantageous to try and speed up the process at any time. Instead, an attitude of acceptance that labour will establish when it is ready, provided that there are no inhibiting factors present, may give the best long term outcome.

When labour is induced

If the labour has been induced, then she will be feeling strong, consistent contractions at frequent intervals from the start. The sudden onset of contractions after a drip of oxytocin has been started gives little time for adjustment to the nature and pace of the resulting labour. In addition, there can be anxiety about what will happen and perhaps concern about being able to cope. As a result, many women request pain killing drugs to reduce the pain of the relentless flow of stong contractions. There is much you can do to ease her discomfort.

- Help her into a comfortable, upright position and keep her as mobile as possible. The drip can be placed on a moveable stand so she can walk around.
- Use all the strategies outlined above to increase her privacy and sense of security.
- Water and heat in the form of showers or hot packs can still be offered.
- Ask if she can labour in the room where she will give birth. Avoid staying in the 'induction' room for longer than necessary.
- Fetal monitoring equipment is often used to check on the baby's reactions to the labour. This can be used intermittently if all is well, and need not be attached continually. There is also no need to lie down if fetal monitoring equipment is being used, and she can sit, stand or walk around near the machine.
- Keep her feeling positive and reassure her about the baby's wellbeing. Once the labour becomes established, the endorphins will begin to be released which will give her some natural protection from the pain of contractions and increase her feeling of being able to cope with the labour.

13

Further ideas for partners and support people

As well as the suggestions already mentioned for making labour easier for your partner, there are other points that should be considered.

Making your needs known in labour

It has often been said that unless you are assertive during labour and birth, then the system will take over and the birth experience will turn out differently from what you were expecting. It is true that unless you make your needs known, those around you, particularly hospital staff whom you have just met, will find it difficult to provide the assistance you require. Many women have felt after the birth that the experience was less than satisfying: things were done that they didn't want; medical management was given precedence over personal wishes; those attending didn't listen to what was being asked. Support people too have often felt that they were pushed aside, their efforts were misunderstood and that situations developed beyond their control, that affected the birth and perhaps even the baby.

You can reduce the chance of these things happening if you have done your 'homework' during the pregnancy, made a careful choice of doctor and hospital, and discussed your preferences well in advance of the labour. It will also help if you can clearly state your questions and requests in labour. You, as a support person, will be the one to speak on the mother's behalf when necessary: to convey her needs, protect her rights and ensure that nothing is done without her consent.

No woman in labour should have to be assertive. The nature of the birth process is such that as the labour hormones begin to flow she will be unable to think clearly, make rational choices or even communicate effectively. If she does attempt these things, then the natural release of hormones will be interrupted and as a result, the birth may be longer, more difficult and more painful than it should be. The labouring mother must be allowed to get on with her task of giving birth without outside interference of any kind. She can be assertive during the pregnancy and will again take an active role in determining her care after the birth, but during labour she must be left in peace to labour as her body dictates. Therefore, her support people, partner, midwife and doctor must use her predetermined birth plan, her expressed wishes and then intuitive common sense to make sure that she gives birth as she wants and finds necessary.

Although much can be decided in advance (and her wishes can be entered onto her medical record in the form of a birth plan or letter from the doctor) it is quite likely that when you arrive at the hospital you will find yourselves being attended by midwives who are complete strangers. You need to get them quickly on side and explain what you want early so that no confusion develops and clear communication lines exists between you. To help you do this you should consider the following.

- Make at least one visit to the labour ward in advance to meet staff and determine hospital policy and procedures.
- When you arrive in labour, take a copy of the birth plan or the letter from her doctor with you and request that it be attached to the nursing notes. This will ensure that all staff, including those who arrive with the next shift, will have a clear understanding of the mother's wishes.
- When you meet the midwife who will be with you for the labour, request her help and outline your plans verbally. You need this midwife as an ally to ensure that hospital routines are avoided and personal preferences, especially in second stage, are observed.
- Be aware of the language you use when speaking to the staff. Loud demands, angry tones and unrealistic requests will all arouse hostility. Remember that these people are there to help you—they need to know what help you require. A polite but firm request will usually be readily accepted, especially if you acknowledge the midwife's unique position in being able to help you with your goals. For example, the requests below are phrased to encourage co-operation:

'We are planning for the birth to go in a certain way. Can you help us to achieve this?'
or
'We know that certain hospital rules generally apply here, but if my partner doesn't specifically need these we want to avoid

them as much as possible. Will you please ask before doing any routine procedures?'
or
'We will need a clear explanation of any medical procedure before it is carried out and time to consider its advantages and disadvantages. Please come back when we have had a chance to talk.'
or
'My partner will find it difficult to answer questions or make decisions as her labour gets stronger. She wants me to act on her behalf so she can be disturbed as little as possible. Please direct your questions to me first.'
or
'We have discussed our preferences for second stage with the doctor and he has agreed that he will follow my partner's wishes at that time. Will you please remind the doctor of this if we are too busy at the time?'

It may seem difficult to be assertive at a time when you are feeling vulnerable and insecure in an unfamiliar hospital setting. If you remember that your partner is relying on you to protect her from disturbance during labour then you will have some incentive to try to provide her with the right environment. The staff and your doctor are there to help you, to provide a service and to make this experience a memorable, personal event. They can do this only if you tell them what you want and how you want things to go—they can't read your mind! They are ordinary people doing a job and have expertise in that area just as you have expertise in your chosen work or profession. Good communication and honest openness will always make for a better psychological and emotional outcome and clear observance of the natural birth process will be better for the baby and the mother.

Handling the hospital stay

Sometimes problems can occur during the post-natal stay in hospital that can take the shine off an otherwise good birth experience. The most common general complaint about maternity services is that following the birth mothers are bombarded with conflicting advice on babycare and breastfeeding at a time when they are easily confused, vulnerable, tired and firmly in a 'patient' role. Everyone seems to have the 'best' advice on how to breastfeed, burp, hold, bath, change nappies and get babies to sleep, including the midwives in the hospital, and visiting friends and relatives. Sometimes the mother is affected by the 'third day blues', a common reaction to the change in hormones after the pregnancy, and these feelings of mild depression and weepiness make coping with the first few days in hospital even more difficult.

You can offer helpful support to your partner at this time. Consider limiting the visitors, or have them come together for a 'party' rather than in smaller groups. If the hospital has an open visiting policy then, unless you set some guidelines for visitors, they will visit at all hours, which can be exhausting. It might be worth asking your friends to visit at home later when you have had time to settle in and feel more confident with the baby.

Try to spend as much time as possible with her during the day while she is in hospital. These first few days are very important in establishing your relationship with the baby and for gaining confidence in caring for your child. You will both be learning how to bathe, change and settle the baby and these will be useful skills for you to know when you are all at home later. Don't be afraid to handle and cuddle your baby—fathers and other close friends are important for your child, who needs close contact with various people to develop social habits.

Breastfeeding takes time to establish, and you will play an important role in helping its success. Protect your partner from unwanted negative comment and support her wishes about breastfeeding and babycare. Once again, she needs to trust her instincts in these areas and this is easier if the environment is secure and peaceful and protected from unwarranted intrusion by others with unhelpful advice.

She may be very hungry after the birth: lactation uses extra energy and hospital menus are not always to everyone's liking. You can bring in additional foods from home to supplement her diet.

Returning home

When you take your partner and new baby home from hospital it will take a few days for you all to settle into a new routine. The household will now revolve around the baby rather than yourselves and many of your standards and expectations about housework, meals, chores and management decisions will have to change. The roles you have both developed within your relationship may also change and these can add to the stresses of the inevitable upheaval in your daily routines. In time, new patterns will emerge as you develop as a family.

If both of you are already familiar with stress management techniques these will be useful right now. You will recognise the physical and emotional changes that are precipitated by stress and will have learned how to recognise and deal with them. If you have never been stressed in this way before (and many parents will never experience anything quite like the stress of bringing home the first baby again!) the following suggestions might be useful.

- Recognise that the major changes you are undergoing at this time are normal, and in many ways to be expected. Nothing can prepare you either for the total commitment a new baby demands or the sudden alterations in your lifestyle. Things will improve in time and eventually you will be able to look back and feel satisfied that you were able to survive and even draw positive strengths from the experience.

- Look for any short cuts and labour saving ideas that you can find to reduce the household chores to a minimum. Caring for the baby and feeding yourselves are the major priorities. Cleaning, entertaining, fancy cooking etc are of lesser importance for the time being and you should not allow them to sap your energies.

- Accept all offers of help, especially of pre-cooked meals or offers of cleaning. When visitors arrive, have them make the tea or coffee and ask them to bring the cake. You should not have to entertain others, especially in the first few weeks. Live-in help (usually offered by a relative) can work well provided that it is understood that the assistance is for household tasks and not care of the baby, which is the mother's right unless she asks for help with this.

- Allow yourselves some time together if you can, and also schedule some time on your own away from the family. This is especially important for a new mother, if she is to avoid burn-out and retain some sense of her personal identity. Motherhood is a twenty-four-hour job, and every mother needs a regular break to recoup energies and pursue personal activities.

- A young baby is easily transportable, so schedule some outings as a family. Try casual rather than strictly timetabled events to avoid feeling pressured. All you will need, especially if the baby is breastfed, are some changes of nappies, and the baby's lambskin or a possum pouch for sleeping. A stroller, pram or possum pouch will be needed if you will be on foot, or a secure baby capsule for the car.

Unexpected outcomes

Sometimes the birth will not have turned out as you had hoped or expected. Perhaps the labour was complicated by a medical emergency, your baby became distressed or sick, or the worst occurred and your baby has died or been born with a handicap. These kinds of events are shattering in their effects on you and your family, and it will take a long time to overcome the inevitable grief. If you now find yourself in one of these situations you will both need time and help to resolve the feelings that result and perhaps the physical trauma that has occurred. It might help you at this time if you can follow any of the suggestions outlined below.

- Understand that the emotional reactions and physical symptoms you are feeling are normal in these circumstances. They are part of the grieving process and the enormous stress these situations impose. Allow yourself time to work through reaction so that it can be fully acknowledged and satisfactorily resolved.
- Talk about what has happened with those who were with you, medical staff, family, social workers or bereavement counsellors, anyone who will listen and accept your reactions as normal.
- You will have many questions to ask and some of these may have no answers. Keep seeking the information you need until you feel satisfied that you know all there is to know. You may need to seek specialist opinions, to have access to your medical records or to seek an independent person to act for you.
- Finding others who have been through a similar experience can be a valuable source of support and insight. They will have much to offer—practical help and suggestions, further information and a truly empathetic listening ear, having been through it themselves. There are support organisations for bereaved parents and parents of handicapped children and these groups often have counsellors available as well.
- Finding another doctor and hospital can be helpful for the next pregnancy. A fresh view, a different approach and an attitude that is not coloured by the last birth experience can make a big difference in getting a better birth next time. This is especially true if you have had a caesarian section or medical intervention that you felt was unwarranted at the time. The section at the beginning of this book on choosing a doctor and seeking a second opinion will give you some guidance on how to change doctors next time.

14

Some final thoughts

It will take time to accept, assimilate and perhaps understand the events surrounding your baby's birth. The hormones released during labour tend to dull the memory and perceptions of labour. Coming to terms with the overall experience is important, to help put into perspective this aspect of femininity and to resolve the various feelings and emotions surrounding birth. It may take a while for this to happen, and as the new mother is working through it all, you, as her partner, can help her in several ways.

- Go over the events of labour together. She will enjoy talking about it and will appreciate your impressions of what happened.
- If you are able to make contact with the midwife who was with you during the labour, she will be happy to fill in any details you want clarified. It would be easiest to do this while you are still in the hospital.
- If you had other support people with you, allow them time to talk over the events too. This kind of debriefing is valuable for everyone concerned.
- If your other children were at the birth of their new sibling, allow them an opportunity to talk about what they saw and felt and to ask any questions they might have.

  Drawing pictures is a good way of assessing their reactions. Giving your older children specific jobs to help you with the baby, accepting their inevitable reactions to the new baby, and providing lots of loving cuddles and reassurance will also help to reduce sibling rivalry.
- When you visit the doctor for your six week check up, ask any questions you still have about the medical management of the labour. Ask for a copy of your file if you wish.
- Writing out an account of the birth is helpful for many women and provides a tangible record for the future. It is best to do this within a week or two of the birth before some of the details fade from memory.

- A letter to the hospital can be an effective way of voicing your feelings about the services offered. Praise those things that you found made your labour and birth more pleasant and effective: positive feedback will encourage the staff to provide the same for others. If you were unhappy about some aspects of your stay, state these clearly (try to avoid emotional overtones), pointing out your reasons for complaint and where the services did not live up to your expectations. A copy of your letter should be sent to the Hospital Board, the Medical Superintendent and the Director of Nursing. Some States also have a Medical Complaints Tribunal that will hear your complaint.

The birth of your baby has been a special time in your lives. Labour is an intense, emotional experience that opens new perspectives on many aspects of life itself. You have come through this experience together and will have discovered much about your relationships, your strengths and yourselves as people. There are many years ahead of child raising that will give you further opportunities for personal development (as well as joys and frustrations!) and once again, your instincts and insights into what feels right for you and your child will be your best guide to parenting. Child rearing is often just as unpredictable as this birth has been. Having come through the challenge of birth together, your roles as parents have begun. Draw strength from your experiences so far, and enjoy the special pleasures your child will give you.

Further reading

The following books will provide you with additional information that will complement this book.

Robertson, Andrea *Preparing for Birth* Sydney: Allen & Unwin, 1989

Odent, Michel *Birth Reborn* London: Century Hutchinson, 1984

Balaskas, Janet *The New Active Birth* Sydney: Allen & Unwin, 1989

Panuthos, Claudia *Transformation through birth* Massachusetts: Bergin and Garvey, 1984

Nancy Cohen and Lois Estner *Silent Knife* Massachusetts: Bergin and Garvey, 1983

Kitzinger, Sheila *Pregnancy and Childbirth* London: Michael Joseph, 1980

Inch, Sally *Birthrights* London: Merlin Press, 1989